Maurice Barry

Clinical Practice in Rheumatology

Foreword by
Professor Michael Doherty

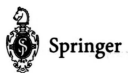

Springer

Maurice Barry, MB, FRCPI
Consultant Rheumatologist
James Connolly Memorial Hospital
Blanchardstown,
Dublin, Ireland

British Library Cataloguing in Publication Data
Barry, Maurice
  Clinical practice in rheumatology
  1. Rheumatology
  I. Title
  616.7′23
ISBN 1852337192

American Library of Congress Cataloging-in-Publication Data
A Catalog record for this book is available from the Library of Congress

ISBN 1-85233-719-2 Springer-Verlag London Berlin Heidelberg

Typeset by Florence Production Ltd, Stoodleigh, Devon, England
Printed at The Cromwell Press, Trowbridge, Wiltshire, England
28/3830–54321 Printed on acid-free paper SPIN 10993811

Dedication

To the patients and staff of the Department
of Rheumatology, Blanchardstown Hospital,
and to Rosie, Rory, Kate and Stevie.

Preface

Rheumatology is predominantly a clinic-based speciality. The medical staff in the clinic often includes doctors in their early postgraduate years who rotate through the specialty every few months. They usually arrive knowing less about the basics of rheumatology than other specialties, but rapidly need to learn what to ask or do next with the patient sitting in front of them. The book is aimed at this group. It will also be of benefit to trainees in general (internal) medicine and general or family practice, and to medical students, rheumatology nurse specialists and allied health professionals. A further aim in writing this book is to reduce the time busy departments need to spend inducting new medical staff every few months.

We have tried to include the curricular requirement in rheumatology likely to be needed for Parts I and II of the Membership in Medicine. Any suggestions for improvements that might be made in future editions are welcome.

Maurice Barry
Consultant Rheumatologist,
James Connolly Memorial Hospital, Dublin

Acknowledgements

The initial draft of some sections was contributed to by junior doctors attached to the team. They include Jillian Drury, Mike McWeeney, Liz Maxwell, Ferga Gleeson and Ai Shiang Bong. Killian O'Rourke and SA Ramakrishnan wrote a number of sections. I thank them for their major contribution to what began as guidelines for use in our department.

Thanks to Sara Tubb for typing the manuscript and to Ray Lohan and Oliver O'Flanagan of the Media Services Department at the Royal College of Surgeons in Ireland for the clinical photographs. Thanks also to those patients who allowed themselves be photographed.

The support of Brenda Dooley of Pharmacia and Melissa Morton and Eva Senior of Springer-Verlag London is much appreciated.

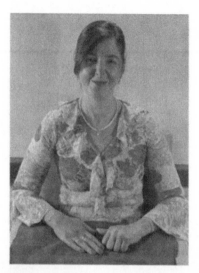

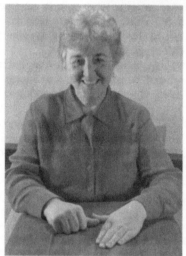 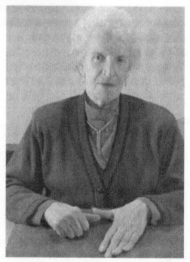

These illustrations show three women with longstanding sero-positive rheumatoid arthritis. They illustrate the reality of recent years for many with rheumatoid arthritis, particularly those treated early and appropriately. Note the absence of ulnar deviation, swan-neck, Boutonniere, Z thumb or other deformities (permissions received).

Foreword

Locomotor assessment is a required competance of any doctor due to the high prevalence of musculoskeletal conditions. The spectrum of these conditions ranges from relatively minor self-limiting mechanical strains to complex life-threatening multisystem disease. This wide range of conditions and the anatomical complexity of the system make clinical assessment of a patient with musculoskeletal symptoms a daunting challenge for many trainees. Often the challenge is made greater because of low prioritisation of musculoskeletal clinical skills teaching in some Medical Schools.

This short handbook, therefore, is very welcome. Written by Maurice Barry a Consultant Rheumatologist in Dublin, it briefly summarises the key practical points relating to the assessment, investigation and management of patients with musculoskeletal disease. Its uncluttered bullet-pointed format and clarity of style make it a rapid and easy source of clinically relevant information. Apart from system-specific detail there is an appropriate emphasis on the wider holistic assessment of the individual with musculoskeletal pain.

This first Edition is fully up-to-date and should prove invaluable to its target audience of Senior House Officers and Specialist Registrars in Rheumatology and General Internal Medicine. It is likely to become the standard Departmental Manual for many UK Rheumatology Units. The book should also prove useful for a wider range of doctors in Primary and Secondary Care and for Allied Health Professionals who work in a Rheumatology Multidisciplinary Team.

Michael Doherty
Professor of Rheumatology
Nottingham University Medical School.

Contents

Rheumatological Disorders

Note to the Reader

A couple of points are worth emphasising:

- Although we treat some interesting and complex diseases, chronic musculoskeletal pain is frequently either caused by or exacerbated by psychosocial distress. If you learn to distinguish the often subtle differences between organic and non-organic causes of pain and can deal capably and sensitively with both, you will enjoy the specialty.
- Be positive with the patient. Making people feel reassured (usually appropriate irrespective of diagnosis) and engendering a positive attitude (always appropriate) can be as potent as any drug and should be appreciated for their true worth.

Before starting the rheumatology rotation you should revise musculoskeletal anatomy; undergraduate orthopaedic and immunology notes should also be revisited.

Glossary of Frequently Used Terms

Arthralgia	*Joint pain, usually with stiffness*
Arthritis	*Joint pain, stiffness and swelling (swelling may be fluid, soft tissue or bony)*
Oligoarthritis	*Arthropathy of 2–4 joints; 5 joints + upwards = polyarthritis. Oligoarthritis and pauci-articular are effectively synonomous*
Synovitis	*Clinical definition is joint soft tissue swelling and tenderness (the hallmark of inflammatory arthritis)*
Tenosynovitis	*Inflammation of a tendon sheath. Presents clinically as linear swelling along a tendon, sometimes with crepitus*
Serositis	*Inflammation of pericardium, pleura or peritoneum (see systemic lupus erythematosus, page 72)*
Spondylosis	*Osteoarthritis of the spine with disc degeneration*
Spondylitis	*Inflammation of the spine*
Spondylolisthesis	*Forward displacement of one vertebra on another*
Spondylolysis	*Congenital or traumatic break in the pars interarticularis of a vertebra; if bilateral can cause a spondylolisthesis*
Subluxation	*Joint surfaces not fully in contact with one another. It is the same as partial dislocation (a term used when due to trauma)*
Sprain	*Acute traumatic injury to a ligament*

History Taking

For new patients, record the history as suggested below. For return patients follow the sequence in Chapter 4 (Clinic Checklist).

New Patients

- Document the patient's presenting symptoms.
- Always relate symptoms to functional difficulty – is there anything they find a bit difficult, very difficult or impossible to do as a result of their symptoms?
- Ask about symptoms associated with rheumatic diseases (see extra-articular symptom review)
- **Treatment history**: Current and tried medications and other treatments (conventional and complementary), history of vaccination (e.g. Reactive arthralgia/arthritis may follow Hepatitis B vaccination). Ask about side effects of therapy.
- **Past history**: Document any previous illnesses. If no apparent problems, ask if they ever took a prescribed medication and document why. Any history of Infection, trauma, Tick-bite (Lyme disease), Transfusion (Hepatitis, HIV) and Travel should be enquired about (ITTTT).
- **Social history**: Ask about the effects of their symptoms on their work and home life. Try to get a sense of whether or not psychosocial distress is contributing to the clinical picture. Is the patient a "worrier"? Do they seem stressed, anxious, depressed? Do they have difficulty relaxing or sleeping? Take an alcohol and smoking history.
- **Family history**: Ask about family history of arthritis and age of onset. Gout, primary osteoarthritis and spondylarthropathies are more likely to be inherited than other arthropathies. Rheumatoid arthritis and connective tissue diseases are less likely to be inherited.

Extra-articular Symptom Review

In all but the most localised rheumatological disorders, enquire about the extra-articular symptoms listed on the manikin below, starting with the hands and finishing with the feet.

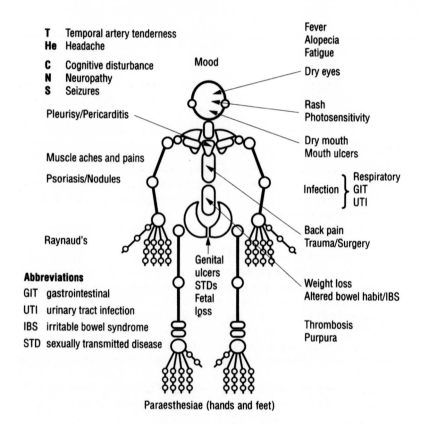

T	Temporal artery tenderness
He	Headache
C	Cognitive disturbance
N	Neuropathy
S	Seizures

Mood

Pleurisy/Pericarditis

Muscle aches and pains

Psoriasis/Nodules

Raynaud's

Fever
Alopecia
Fatigue

Dry eyes

Rash
Photosensitivity

Dry mouth
Mouth ulcers

Respiratory
Infection } GIT
UTI

Back pain
Trauma/Surgery

Genital
ulcers
STDs
Fetal
loss

Weight loss
Altered bowel habit/IBS

Thrombosis
Purpura

Abbreviations

GIT	gastrointestinal
UTI	urinary tract infection
IBS	irritable bowel syndrome
STD	sexually transmitted disease

Paraesthesiae (hands and feet)

Locomotor Examination 2

There are more than 100 joints in the body, not to mention muscles, tendons and other soft tissue structures. Some joints are superficial and easy to examine, others like hips and sacroiliac joints are deep and difficult to assess. The same severity of disease (e.g. in Rheumatoid arthritis) will produce very different clinical findings in an MCP joint (swelling/deformity) compared with a hip (usually no swelling/deformity).

Careful locomotor examination is therefore time-consuming and difficult. To improve efficiency in the assessment of the locomotor system, consider locomotor examination to consist of three levels of increasing complexity:

- gait, arms, leg, spine (GALS)
- joint examination
- clinical signs of specific conditions or diseases

The GALS examination may be sufficient in general (internal) medicine clinics but patients attending rheumatology clinics need more detailed examination.

GALS Examination

This is a screening examination for locomotor abnormality. It helps to answer the question: Is there a significant locomotor disorder? It does not give a diagnosis but may point towards one. The screening examination is limited and could, for example, completely miss a problem such as severe tennis elbow.

Most of the screening examination is done without touching the patient. It is easiest if the examiner demonstrates the movement and the patient follows it.

Gait

- Watch the patient walking. Look for loss of symmetry, stiffness and difficulty walking, use of aids, difficulty with transfers, etc.

3

Arms

- With the patient sitting in front of you, observe the hands supinated and pronated
- Ask the patient to make a fist and then pinch the tip of the index and middle finger to the thumb
- Ask the patient to flex and extend the elbows
- Place the hands behind head with elbows as far back as possible (full external rotation and abduction of shoulder)
- Ask the patient to place the hands behind their back with thumb pointing upwards (full internal rotation of shoulder)
- Look for asymmetry, loss of movement or facial wincing

Spine

- With the patient seated in front of you, ask the patient to bend the neck from side to side. Look for pain and /or restriction
- Ask the patient to stand up and inspect the whole spine from behind and from the side. Look for deformity
- Ask the patient to bend forward at the hips with straight knees. Look for ease of movement and symmetry

Legs

- Position the patient on a couch/bed, reclining comfortably
- Look for asymmetry and /or wasting
- Inspect feet for swelling, deformity or callosity
- Ask the patient to bend each knee up in turn. Watch for ease, restriction of movement and for any pain
- Hold the knee and hip in 90° flexion and internally rotate the hip. Following this rotate the hip externally. Compare with other side and watch for restriction or discomfort
- Extend the knee with one hand on the knee joint and feel for crepitus
- Palpate the knee for warmth or swelling
- Record any abnormalities found. Some departments use a manikin to facilitate this

Joint Examination

The examination of individual joints involves the following principles:

- look
- feel
- move
- measure
- compare

This level of examination applies to any symptomatic joint or where an abnormality has been identified by the GALS examination. The rheumatology department should demonstrate the technique of individual joint examination when you start the rotation.

For any symptomatic joint:

- Look for:
  - erythema
  - scars
  - rashes
  - swelling
  - deformity
  - subluxation
  - muscle wasting
- Feel for:
  - warmth
  - tenderness
  - soft and spongy swelling (synovitis)
  - fluctuant swelling (effusion)
  - bony swelling
  - crepitus
- Move:
  - passive movements (examiner moves the joint)
  - active movement (patient moves the joint)
  - assess stability of joints
- Measure:
  - range of movements (see below)
  - muscle bulk
  - spinal movements
- Compare:
  - all of the above with other side where relevant.

Clinical Signs of Specific Conditions or Diseases

The clinical features of many specific conditions are covered in Chapter 3 (Common New Presentations) and also under individual subject headings.

The signs are best learnt in the clinic, as they will soon be forgotten if seen only in a book.

In summary, follow the basic principles of rheumatological examination as outlined. For all but the most straightforward of conditions, e.g. tennis elbow, all systems should be examined in addition to the locomotor system. For detailed description of individual joint examination and signs of specific conditions see the list of further reading.

Range of Movement (ROM)

Two issues commonly surface:

Do You Assess Active Movement, Passive Movement or Both?

Most rheumatologists primarily assess passive movement unless a joint is acutely tender. The overall examination is a mixture of both, e.g. spinal movement is primarily active, hip examination mostly passive. Learn the techniques in the clinic.

How Do You Document Restriction of Movement?

Few rheumatologists record joint ROM in degrees. ROM often varies with time of day (e.g. spinal movement improves during the day) and use of NSAIDS on that day. There is also considerable inter-observer variability so comparisons may be meaningless unless performed by the same observer. Describing the effect of limitation in terms of functional impairment (e.g. eating, dressing, walking) is more important.

- Record whether limitation of ROM is mild, moderate or severe (dividing normal ROM for that joint into thirds) and whether limitation is due to pain or mechanical restriction
- For larger joints limitation of movement in a key direction may be recorded in degrees, e.g. elbow or knee lacking full extension by 10°
- If limitation is not passively correctable it is usually called a fixed deformity, e.g. elbow lacking full extension by 10° = fixed flexion deformity of 10°
- If range of movement is restricted equally actively and passively, the restriction is usually articular in origin
- If passive range of movement is greater than active range of movement then soft tissue origin is likely (e.g. tendonitis)

Resisted Movement

Active movement by patient to which the examiner applies a counteractive force, useful for assessing tendinopathies (e.g. rotator cuff tendonitis, epicondylitis).

PLATES

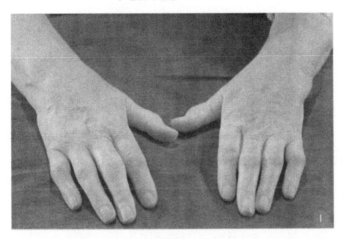

Plate I – Active rheumatoid arthritis. Prominent symmetrical PIP joint swelling. A reduction in the number and depth of normal skin indentations over the joints indicates soft tissue swelling. When accompanied by tenderness, this soft tissue swelling is called synovitis.

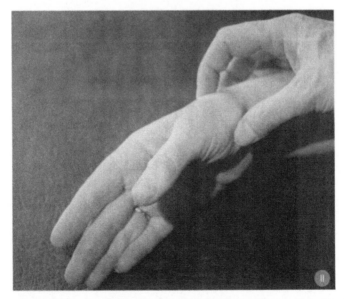

Plate II – Osteoarthritis of the first carpometacarpal joint. Bony swelling results in prominence and increased breadth of the joint. A typical feature of hand osteoarthritis along with DIP and PIP joint swelling, but often missed.

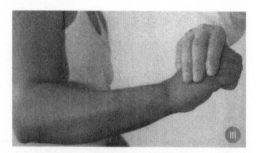

Plate III – Resisted extension of the wrist. The patient attempts to extend the wrist against resistance. Pain felt at the lateral epicondyle (not wrist) with this manoeuvre suggests lateral epicondylitis. Tenderness over the lateral epicondyle itself is less specific.

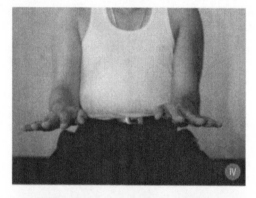

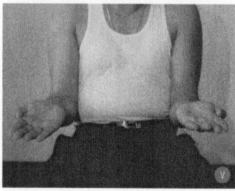

Plates IV and V – Active pronation (IV) and supination (V). Disease of superior or inferior radioulnar joint or both (e.g. in inflammatory arthritis) will cause restriction of movement. Note elbows held at sides to exclude shoulder rotation.

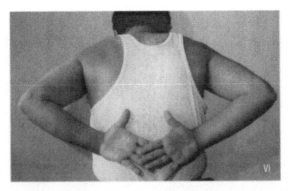

Plate VI – Active shoulder movement. A combination of internal rotation, extension and adduction. If this manoeuvre and placing hands behind head (abduction and external rotation) are full and pain free, significant shoulder disease is unlikely.

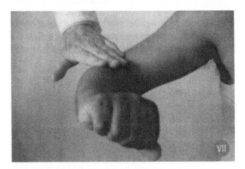

Plate VII –Resisted abduction of the shoulder. The patient attempts to abduct the shoulder against resistance. Pain felt in the deltoid region is seen in rotator cuff and specifically supraspinatus tendonitis.

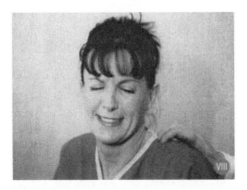

Plate VIII –Muscle tenderness associated with fibromyalgia.

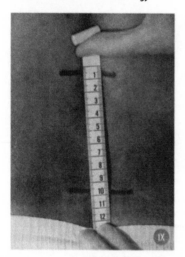 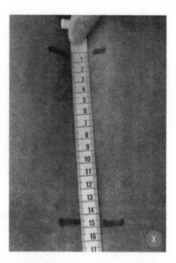

Plates IX and X – Schobers test: measures lumbar spine flexion. Make two marks with the patient erect, one at the "dimples of Venus" – the posterior superior iliac spines – and another 10 cm above. The distance between the marks should increase by at least 5 cm on spinal flexion.

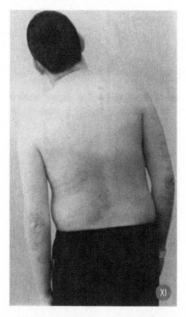

Plate XI – Restriction of lateral flexion of the spine is an early feature of spondylitis. In this case the spondylitis is secondary to psoriasis (note rash over extensor surfaces of the elbows).

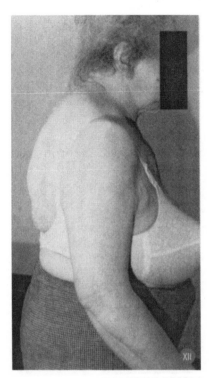

Plate XII – Dorsal kyphosis in a woman with osteoporosis and vertebral fractures. Treatment at this stage is of limited benefit. The key to successful management is recognition of risk factors for osteoporosis and early intervention to prevent fractures.

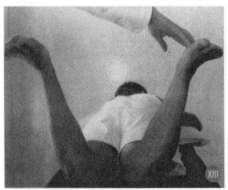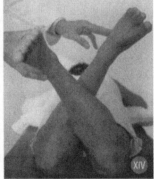

Plates XIII and XIV – Internal (XIII) and external (XIV) rotation of the hips in the prone position. Useful for comparing one hip with the other and for detecting early hip disease.

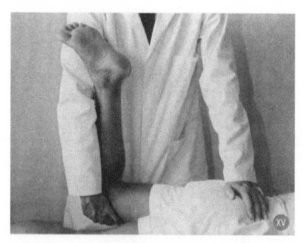

Plate XV – Hip extension in the prone position. Hip extension combined with maximal knee flexion (not shown here) is a femoral nerve stretch test.

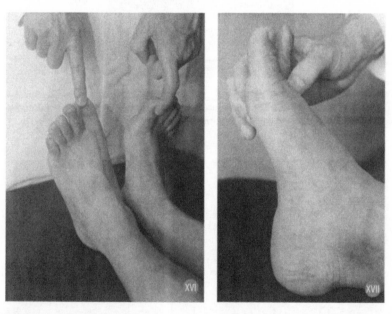

Plate XVI – Weakness of dorsiflexion of the great toe (in this case the left). A typical motor feature of L5 root lesions.

Plate XVII – Palpating individual MTP joints for swelling and tenderness. MTP joint involvement is a typical early feature of rheumatoid arthritis.

The diagnosis in many patients can be made on the history and examination alone. Much is due to pattern recognition, i.e. a combination of typical symptoms and clinical signs coming together. Below is a list of the locomotor symptoms and clinical signs of some common rheumatological disorders.

PIP Joint Pain

- Age 40+, female + bony swelling → osteoarthritis (OA)
- Any age, soft tissue swelling and tenderness → synovitis? cause → symmetry → rule out rheumatoid arthritis (RA)
- Asymmetric – consider spondylarthropathy, e.g. psoriatic or reactive arthritis

MCP Soft Tissue Swelling and Tenderness

- Synovitis → symmetry → rule out RA
- Asymmetric – consider spondylarthropathy especially if digital swelling (dactylitis) present

Thumb Base Pain

- Age 40+, female + bony swelling 1st carpometacarpal CMC → 1st CMC OA
- Consider De Quervain's tenosynovitis

Elbow Pain

Lateral Aspect

- Tender lateral epicondyle + pain on resisted extension wrist → lateral epicondylitis

Medial Aspect

- Tender medial epicondyle and pain on resisted flexion wrist → medial epicondylitis

Over Olecranon Process

- Local soft tissue swelling → olecranon bursitis (other possibilities gouty tophi or rheumatoid nodules)

Upper Arm Pain (see also "Shoulder Pain")

- Pain on reaching behind, lifting arm, shoulder sore to lie on, ↓ active ROM in rotation → likely shoulder origin
- Pain on resisted movement → likely rotator cuff disorder
- Marked ↓ active and passive ROM → adhesive capsulitis
- If shoulder appears normal examine neck, supraclavicular fossae, chest and axillae (large differential diagnosis)

Trapezius Pain

- Tender acromioclavicular (AC) joint → AC joint origin
- Chronic pain associated with widespread pain and muscle tenderness → fibromyalgia
- ↓ ROM neck → may be cervical in origin (especially if asymmetric)

Thoracic Spine Pain

- Young, prominent stiffness, ↓ ROM, ↓ chest expansion → ankylosing spondylitis likely
- Older, dorsal kyphosis → osteoporotic vertebral fractures likely
- Consider intrathoracic causes
- In all with thoracic pain ensure FBC, ESR, bone profile, plain radiographs normal

Anterior Chest Wall Pain

- Tender only over individual costo-hondral junctions → costochondritis
- Diffusely tender → rule out fibromyalgia

Low Back Pain

Acute

- Likely lumbar, mechanical
- Disc or facet joint

Chronic

- Young, widespread pain + tender points → fibromyalgia
- Chronic, with sciatica (see definition) → disc protrusion
- Chronic, 60+ with buttock pain worse on exertion, radiates to legs → rule out spinal stenosis
- Consider intra-abdominal causes

Lateral Hip Pain

- 40 +, sore to lie on, tenderness localised to greater trochanter → trochanteric bursitis

Pain in Groin or Anterior Thigh

- Pain on hip movement, ↓ ROM → hip origin → most commonly OA
- Hip movement normal → large differential; consider high lumbar disc, femoral neuropathy, diabetic amyotrophy; meralgia paraesthetica (compression lat. cutaneous nerve of thigh) abdominal source, hernia, saphena varix, knee origin; also pelvic fracture, Paget's disease, bone secondaries in older people
- Needs careful assessment
- Check FBC, ESR, bone profile, appropriate radiographs

Knee Pain

Anterior

- Patellar abnormality – hypermobility, tracking, chondromalacia, osteoarthritis
- Anterior swelling and tenderness – pre- or infrapatellar bursitis

Diffuse

- Bony periarticular swelling → OA
- Synovitis (↑ heat, effusion, soft tissue swelling)
- Trauma or sudden onset → ligament or meniscal injury

Ankle Pain

Posterior

- Achilles swollen, tender → Achilles tendonitis or Achilles bursitis
- Dip in Achilles tendon → consider unrecognised Achilles tear

Anterior/Lateral/Medial

- Tenosynovitis (lateral = peroneal, medial = tibialis posterior)
- Synovitis (↑ heat, diffuse soft tissue swelling, tenderness)
- Soft tissue injury/sprain
- Hypermobility

Heel Pain

- Heel tenderness with associated spondylarthropathy → plantar fasciitis
- Tenderness only → fat pad syndrome

Foot Pain

- Acute, swelling, redness → rule out gout
- Diffuse, chronic → rule out pes planus
- 1st mtp, chronic → bony swelling → OA
- Swelling of a toe ± redness → likely dactylitis (see spondy-larthropathies)
- Symmetrical MTP pain, swelling and tenderness → rule out RA

Practice Point

It is not uncommon to find patients presenting with widespread symptoms who have a multiplicity of local conditions, e.g. 55-year-old woman with hand, shoulder and foot symptoms. Examination may demonstrate carpal tunnel syndrome, left rotator cuff tendonitis and 1st MTP OA.

In acute monoarthritis the working diagnosis is septic arthritis until proven otherwise by negative Gram stain and culture of an aspirate unless clinical pattern is classical e.g. acute 1st MTP gout (podagra).

Clinic Checklist 4

The clinic visit of each patient should be documented in the following sequence. This applies to return and new patients. For new patients, diagnosis is replaced by a detailed history (see Chapter 1, History Taking).

1 **Diagnosis:** Write it down when it is definite or else document the features if there is any uncertainty about diagnosis e.g. rash, ESR ↑, ANA strong positive? SLE. Document disease duration
2 **Current treatment** and any significant side effects
3 **Medical** conditions of relevance
4 **Current symptoms** or main problem – compare progress to previous visit. Are they better/worse/same?
5 **Examination:** Document findings and the relevant positives and negatives
6 **Results** of recent investigations
7 **Assessment** (commit yourself)
   — inflammatory or mechanical problems
   — bone/joint/soft tissue in origin
   — your global assessment of severity
8 Outline **plan** (discuss where uncertain)
9 **Discussion** with patient (information, reassurance, etc.)
10 Give **prescription**, where appropriate, to last at least until next visit
11 Give **forms** for blood tests, radiographs, etc. where appropriate
12 **Letter** to referring doctor or family practitioner using above structure. If the rheumatologist or speciality trainee saw the patient with you, state this in the letter.

Practice Point

If there is any uncertainty about what medication patients are taking, staple a note to their appointment card reminding them to bring all tablets on their next visit.

Common Operational Issues   **5**

All rheumatology departments operate in slightly different ways. The following questions (among others) arise with every medical staff changeover. Encouraging your departmental head to produce written guidelines will save incoming doctors having to find the answers to the same questions.

- What is the procedure if the patient doesn't want to see you but wants the rheumatologist?
- Is patient or their family doctor routinely contacted about test results (normal or abnormal) or must they wait until their next clinic visit? (potentially months away) Who contacts them?
- What is done about patients (a) new, (b) return, who don't turn up? What are your responsibilities in this regard?
- What information is contained in the (a) clinic letter, (b) discharge letter?
- What happens when (a) the family doctor, or (b) the patient rings you for a sooner appointment?
- Can patients without a follow-up appointment make further appointments themselves?
- When is the next routine new/return appointment?
- Who is responsible for disease modifying anti-rheumatic drugs (DMARDs) monitoring – hospital, family doctor or shared?

Imaging Guidelines   6

- Doctors new to rheumatology almost always over-order plain radiographs
- Radiographs do not commonly make the diagnosis in rheumatology; it is usually clinical
- Radiographs of most newly painful joints will be unremarkable apart from age-related changes

When to Order Plain Radiographs

- Small joints (hands or feet) in inflammatory arthritis when the presence or severity of erosive changes is in question
- Persisting monoarthritis at presentation (for diagnosis)
- At extended intervals for progression (e.g. 2 years)
- Sacro-iliac joints for diagnosis when spondylarthropathy suspected
- Regional pain, e.g. pelvis, thoracic spine, when diagnosis not clear despite careful history and examination, or for assessment of severity in established disease
- In established joint disease e.g. RA, where individual joint problems are unresponsive to conservative methods, and active intervention e.g. surgery is under consideration

Practice Point

In someone with widespread spinal pain, the likely diagnosis in terms of prevalence is fibromyalgia. Plain radiography of cervical, thoracic and lumbar spine together delivers a radiation dose equivalent to 300 chest radiographs.

Knee Imaging

- Specify weight-bearing views for knee radiographs
- Skyline view where appropriate to assess patella

Nuclear Medicine

- Isotope bone scan may demonstrate or localise joint or bone inflammation/infection not evident clinically or on plain radiograph
- Order in consultation with speciality trainee or rheumatologist

CT Scan

Useful in particular situations:

- lumbar disc protrusion with neurological signs in legs, where surgery contemplated
- older patients with history of spinal claudication to assess presence or severity of lumbar spinal stenosis (again where surgery is contemplated)

Ultrasound

- Operator dependent but can be useful for assessment of soft tissue lesions, e.g. Achilles, plantar fascia, or for monoarticular arthropathy, e.g. hip pain. A technique of increasing clinical utility for both diagnosis and guided injection

MRI Scan

- Useful for assessment of muscle (myositis), joints e.g. shoulder, hip, knee, soft tissue e.g. rotator cuff tear
- Spine – disc protrusion, neurological compromise – either spinal cord or peripheral nerves (but remember – spinal cord ends at L2)
- Discuss with speciality trainee or rheumatologist if you feel MRI scan is indicated

It can be difficult to precisely measure aspects of rheumatic diseases such as impairment in activities of daily living (ADL) or disease activity in a condition involving a number of organ systems, e.g. SLE.

Validated instruments have been developed for use both generally and in individual diseases such as ankylosing spondylitis, SLE and osteoarthritis. They may be particularly useful for comparing new therapies in groups of patients or for following progress in individual patients over a period of time. The extent to which they are used varies from one department to another. Below is a small selection:

SLEDAI	SLE disease activity index (does what it says)
SLICC	SLE index of organ damage
BASDAI	Bath ankylosing spondylitis disease activity index
BASFAI	Bath ankylosing spondylitis functional activity index
HAQ	Health assessment questionnaire. Assesses impairment in activities of daily living, e.g. dressing, eating, walking, etc., and converts this to a number between 0 and 3. Significant difficulty with ADL is associated with score greater than 1.5. Minimum clinically meaningful change is 0.21.
SF36	Short form of 36 questions measures health-related components of quality of life. Tries to help us make treatment decisions in the context of the patient's actual health-related quality of life priorities and not our perception of their priorities.
WOMAC	Measures impact of osteoarthritis (devised in Western Ontario)
HAD	Hospital anxiety and depression scale. Recognises high prevalence of significant (i.e. requiring intervention) anxiety and depression in hospital patients.
AIMS	Arthritis impact measurement scale. Somewhat similar to SF-36 but is specific for those with arthritis.

ACR 20, 50, 70   Index developed by the American College of Rheumatology to assess change in rheumatoid arthritis disease activity in clinical trials, e.g. ACR 20 refers to the percentage of patients achieving a 20% reduction in a defined set of activity measures including number of tender joints (tender joint count – TJC), number of swollen joints (swollen joint count – SJC), etc.

How to Manage Patients 8

General Guidelines

These will vary between departments.

How Often Should Patients be Reviewed?

- Inflammatory arthritis
  - if active - 2–3 months (see section on Inflammatory Arthritis for assessment of activity)
  - if inactive and stable - 6 months+
- Non-inflammatory
  - fibromyalgia - discharge or "open" appointment
  - OA - "open" follow up or 6 months
- Soft tissue problems
  - 3–4 months or discharge, depending on response to treatment

Prescriptions

- Give a minimum of 6 months prescription for DMARD
- Give a new prescription at each clinic visit (so patient, pharmacist and family doctor know what treatment was advised at the last clinic visit)

Who to Admit

Policy will vary depending on local facilities, practice:

- Active inflammatory arthritis with significant disability
- For further investigation to establish diagnosis (complex cases)
- To commence on new disease modifying agent (very selective, but especially older patients)
- Those requiring intensive rehabilitation

Blood Forms

- Give appropriate blood forms until next clinic appointment (unless monitoring is performed by family doctor)
- Bloods are usually checked every 2–3 months while on DMARDS (see drug protocols)
- Need at least monthly bloods for 3 months when commencing DMARDs

When to Seek Advice

Unless all patients are seen by rheumatologist and or speciality trainee:

- Active disease
- No firm diagnosis
- Abnormal investigations (e.g. persisting high ESR 20–30+)
- Lack of response to treatment
- Drug side effects
- Complex problems
- Considering referral to another specialty, e.g. orthopaedics, endocrinology, psychiatry
- Patient appears dissatisfied with the consultation.

The Power of Reassurance

Many patients attending rheumatology clinics have two problems: the first is their symptoms (pain, loss of function, etc.) and the second is their concern about the implications of those symptoms. The second is often of greater importance to the patient but is commonly less well handled (by doctor and patient) than is the first.

Most patients with persisting musculoskeletal pain wonder if they have arthritis. The image of arthritis in the population is of progressive pain, disability and the absence of a cure. It's little wonder, then, that patients arrive with considerable worries about the future. They worry about how they'll be in a few years, about their ability to work or remain independent and if they'll cause more "damage" if they keep going.

The doctor has a crucial role in managing these concerns. Many patients' vision of the future (irrespective of diagnosis) is unduly negative, so it is very important to foster a positive and realistic attitude. Doing this successfully may not be easy and is a communication skill that is often not learnt in medical school. Also, if patients sense that you are not taking their difficulties seriously enough they will not be reassured by what you say and your effectiveness is reduced considerably.

Look at it from the patient's point of view. Telling someone not to worry, it's only early arthritis is not reassuring at all, as their understanding is that it will simply get worse as time goes by. Always ask the patient what worries them most about their problem and then address the issue in a positive way, while recognising their difficulties.

A few common situations where reassurance has a major effect include the following:

- Hand pain in a perimenopausal woman with hand OA. They usually worry about chronic pain, pain spreading to other joints and deformities. The truth is that the pain settles after a couple of years and the bony swellings often become irrelevant to them
- The finding of "arthritis" in the spine on plain radiograph in patients with recent onset neck pain. The "arthritis" is usually incidental and asymptomatic and going to remain so. The neck pain may be postural, stress related or mechanical
- New onset RA. Patients may view the news as catastrophic and see themselves developing deformities, disability and facing a lifetime of pain. The prognosis for new onset RA has improved dramatically in recent years. Patients need to know they are usually unfair on themselves if they foresee a "slippery slope" of deteriorating function and chronic pain

There are many other examples – e.g. lateral epicondylitis, trochanteric bursitis, benign hypermobility, fibromyalgia – where having a diagnosis and understanding the condition are reassuring.

Psychosocial Aspects of Rheumatology

- While chronic psychosocial distress (see "Fibromyalgia") commonly causes musculoskeletal pain, patients who have chronic rheumatic diseases often have problems with:
  - depression and anxiety
  - decreased self-esteem and confidence
  - loss of independence and security in both career and home life
  - increased stress due to social changes and disability
  - fear of becoming physically dependent and disabled
- It is important to be aware of any problems in the patient's work and home life and to look for indications that a patient may be depressed. Sexual problems can be difficult for everyone to talk about but should not be ignored
- Psychiatric consultation and/or anti-depressant medication should be considered in patients who demonstrate signs of depression that interferes with everyday functioning
- Individual, family or group therapy with a psychologist might be also considered. Some rheumatology departments have a clinical psychologist as part of the multidisciplinary team

- All members of the rheumatology team – doctors, ward staff, rheumatology nurse specialist (RNS), physiotherapist, occupational therapist (OT) – have a role in providing support to patients, especially those with chronic disease

Complementary Treatments

Many surveys indicate a high frequency of usage of alternative or complementary treatments in patients with musculoskeletal disorders. It is easy to understand that this happens when some busy doctors prescribe indefinite supplies of potentially toxic drugs that may not work well. Patients often find that alternative treatments work well for them. This could be because of a placebo effect – the patient wants to believe the treatment will work. It could be because the alternative practitioner is empathic and reassuring, and encourages a positive attitude. It could be due to a real but untested effect of the drug, an example of which may be glucosamine and chondroitin sulfate in OA. These were previously deemed to be placebos, but some evidence is accumulating of a true effect in placebo controlled trials.

Commonly encountered therapies include acupuncture, chiropractic manipulation, osteopathy, reflexology, massage, and preparations including herbal remedies, glucosamine, apple cider vinegar, devil's claw and topical procaine.

Doctors' attitudes to such treatments vary. The best approach is to keep an open mind while advocating those treatments in conventional medicine which are of proven benefit. A dismissive attitude to complementary therapies often offends patients and can reduce your effectiveness.

Analgesics

- The first drug for most musculoskeletal pain should be **paracetamol**
- Chronic pain with inflammation often responds well to NSAIDs (see below)
- Compound analgesics containing paracetamol or aspirin with a low dose opioid analgesic (e.g. codeine phosphate 8 mg) are commonly used
- Compound analgesics containing a full dose of opioid (e.g. codeine phosphate 30 mg) should be prescribed only with caution, especially in elderly people. Nausea, severe constipation and drowsiness occur quite frequently

Opioid Analgesics

- Repeated administration may cause **physical dependence** (i.e. withdrawal symptoms on sudden cessation) and tolerance. **Tolerance** usually results in increases by ~10% of drug dose per year
- **Addiction** (i.e. compulsive use greatly in excess of recommended doses) is uncommon in chronic pain – less than 10% of patients
- Some doctors undertreat chronic pain because of a fear of patients developing addiction and tolerance, yet the incidence of addiction and tolerance to opioids is low

Codeine

- Effective for mild to moderate pain
- Constipating in long-term use; common compound preparations include (all plus paracetamol):
  — Solpadeine (8 mg) per tablet
  — Solpadol (30 mg) per tablet
  — Tylex (30 mg) per tablet

Dextropropoxyphene

- Less potent than codeine, e.g. (plus paracetamol) co-proxamol

Dihydrocodeine

- Similar to codeine but probably more potent

Oxycodone

- Potent analgesic for moderate pain

Pentazocine

- Partial agonist and antagonist properties. Can produce pain if taken by patients already on other opioids

Tramadol

- For moderate to severe pain
- Reported to have fewer opioid adverse effects
- Less constipation, respiratory depression and addiction potential

Buprenorphine

- Agonist and antagonist properties. Can cause withdrawal when given to patients on other opioids
- Effects only partly reversed by naloxone
- Transdermal patch now available

Fentanyl

- Transdermal patch, changed every 3 days
- Potent, long half-life
- Less addictive, less nausea and less constipating than morphine

Morphine

- Not commonly used in rheumatology

Practice Point

If you prescribe a potent or high-dose opioid, prescribe a laxative in addition. Do not wait for constipation to occur.

Neuropathic Pain

- E.g. postherpetic neuralgia, painful peripheral neuropathy, nerve root irritation
- Amitriptyline, carbamazepine and gabapentin may be useful
- Start with low doses and increase over days to weeks depending on efficiency and tolerability

Non-steroidal Anti-inflammatory Drugs (NSAIDs)

- These agents are indicated for pain and stiffness in inflammatory arthritis or short term and intermittent use in osteoarthritis. They are also widely used in soft tissue conditions, including fibromyalgia. A number of studies have suggested that patients prefer NSAIDs to simple analgesics, even in non-inflammatory conditions.

- Studies comparing NSAIDs have shown equivalence in terms of efficacy, usually when measured over 6–12 weeks of therapy for osteoarthritis. The focus of recent anti-inflammatory drug research has been in improving gastrointestinal tolerability. In recent years two new agents (celecoxib, rofecoxib) offering high levels of gastrointestinal safety have become available. Both drugs are specific inhibitors of cyclo-oxygenase 2 (Cox 2), the form of cyclo-oxygenase of most relevance to inflammation. The lack of inhibition of Cox 1 results in improved tolerability and safety with very low rates of serious upper gastrointestinal adverse events (perforation, ulcer, bleeding) compared with standard NSAIDs.

- Cox 2 specific agents are particularly suited to those requiring an anti-inflammatory agent who have any of the following risk factors:
  - age over 65
  - using concomitant medications likely to increase GI adverse effects (e.g. steroids, warfarin)
  - those requiring prolonged use of maximum dose NSAIDs (e.g. persistent inflammatory arthritis).
  - serious co-morbidity, e.g. diabetes mellitus, renal or hepatic impairment.

- Cox 2 specific agents should be prescribed only with caution in those with a history of peptic ulceration. They are best avoided in those with previous haemorrhage or perforation.

- Many NSAIDs are available. None is unequivocally superior in terms of efficacy. The frequency of adverse reactions – gastrointestinal, hepatic, renal and cardiovascular –associated with each NSAID varies. Prescribing habits among rheumatologists also vary widely.

Disease-modifying Drugs (DMARDs)

Methotrexate (MTX)

Indications

- Used for treatment of active inflammatory arthritis – usually rheumatoid arthritis and psoriatic arthropathy
- Mode of action unknown, slow acting over 4 weeks–4 months

Administration

- Once weekly oral dose
- May be given intramuscularly or subcutaneously if response to oral route insufficient
- Usual dose 7.5–20 mg **weekly**; comes in 2.5 mg or 10 mg tablets
- Folic acid 5 mg the day after MTX reduces GIT side effects
- Give annual influenza vaccine

Side Effects

- Well tolerated overall
- Nausea on day of dosage most common side effect
- Co-prescription of granisetron may overcome this
- Liver
  - may cause abnormal liver function tests (LFTs), especially AST/ALT (SGOT, SGPT)
  - enzyme elevation >3 times baseline is an indication to temporarily withdraw drug
  - lesser abnormalities – can observe – see local protocol
  - persistent LFTs ↑ – liver biopsy may be required
- Lung
  - pneumonitis has been described in 3–4% on MTX, so consider chest radiograph in those who develop respiratory symptoms, e.g. cough, fever, dyspnoea
- Diarrhoea, mouth ulcers, abdominal discomfort – may respond to an increase in folic acid dosage
- Leucopoenia/thrombocytopenia – uncommon
- Teratogenic – should not be used in pregnancy
- Conception should be avoided for 6 months after cessation of treatment in both men and women

Interactions

- Diclofenac (potentiation of MTX effects); trimethoprim (folate antagonism)

* Retinoids (e.g. isotretinoin)
* Alcohol consumption increases risk of toxicity

Safety Monitoring

* FBC and LFTs monthly for first 3 months of therapy and every 2 months afterwards

When to Withhold MTX

* Liver enzymes > 3 times baseline
* Serious concomitant medical illness
* Acute infection
* Acute pulmonary symptoms
* Pregnancy
* Skin rash or oral ulcers
* It is not necessary to stop methotrexate before or after surgery – no evidence of excess infection or delayed wound healing in those remaining on MTX

Sulfasalazine

Indications

* Inflammatory arthritis – RA, psoriatic arthritis, seronegative arthritis
* Onset of action delayed for several weeks to months

Dose

* Start at 500 mg twice daily
* Increase after 1 week to maintenance dose of 1g twice daily

Side Effects

* Nausea, anorexia, headache, mouth ulcers most common
* Some patients report yellow discoloration of skin, urine or contact lenses
* Oligospermia (usually reversible)
* Skin rash
* Alopecia
* Mood – depression, irritability

Drug Monitoring

* FBC and LFTs monthly for 3 months, then every 3 months

When to Stop Treatment

- WCC drops below 4000 (neutrophils < 2000)
- platelets below 100 000
- LFTs > twice normal

Hydroxychloroquine

Indications

- SLE
- RA
- Sjögren's syndrome

Dose

- 200–400 mg daily – do not exceed 6.5 mg/kg (higher doses associated with eye toxicity)

Side Effects

- Rash
- Depigmentation of hair and skin – reversible
- Eyes – retinopathy and corneal deposits (rare if daily dose <6.5 mg/kg)
- Leucopenia
- Thrombocytopenia
- GIT intolerance

Monitoring

- Eyes – ophthalmology review. Need for this is controversial if 6.5 mg/kg per day is not exceeded – see local protocol. Some recommend review only after 5 years of therapy

Azathioprine

Indications

- Connective tissue disease
- RA

Dose

- Maintenance of 100–150 mg daily depending on body weight and hepatic and renal function (maximum 2.5 mg/kg)

- Give annual flu vaccine
- Check for thiopurine *S*-methyltransferase (TPMT) deficiency before starting azathioprine if available locally. Enzyme deficiency inhibits drug metabolism, causing toxicity

Side Effects

- Hypersensitivity (uncommon) → flu-like reaction → discontinue immediately
- GI intolerance
- Increased risk of malignancy with long-term use
- Malaise
- Leucopenia
- Thrombocytopenia

Monitoring

- Monthly FBC and LFTS
- Discontinue therapy if
  — WCC < 4000
  — platelets < 150 000

Avoid

- Allopurinol – inhibits metabolism of azathioprine and may lead to drug toxicity

Gold

Indications

- RA – now rarely used
- Administered as deep intramuscular (IM) injection
- Initially as test dose of 10 mg, followed by 50 mg weekly dose until 1g has been given, then 50 mg IM monthly.

Side Effects

- Itch
- Rash
- Mouth ulcers
- Thrombocytopenia
- Neutropenia
- Pneumonitis
- Proteinuria

- if "trace" on > 2 consecutive occasions, stop! – recheck, restart if absent
- if proteinuria > 1+ persists, stop and do 24-hour urine. If protein loss < 500 mg/24 h, continue cautiously and monitor
- NB: can cause membranous glomerulonephritis

Monitoring

- FBC and urinalysis before each injection

Ciclosporin (Cyclosporin)

Indications

- RA – active despite other DMARDS
- Less commonly used since advent of biologic therapies

Dose

- 2.5–3 mg/kg in divided doses for 6 weeks
- Maintenance – titrate according to efficacy and tolerability up to maximum of 5 mg/kg per day
- Onset of clinical response – 1–3 months
- Give annual flu vaccine

Contraindications

- Impaired renal function
- Uncontrolled hypertension
- Uncontrolled infection
- Malignancy
- Pregnancy and breast-feeding

Side Effects

- Renal toxicity
- Reduce dose if serum creatinine exceeds normal range or increase > 50% of pretreatment levels
- Repeat creatinine 1 week later; if still elevated, stop cyclosporin
- Hypertension
- Liver function – a slight increase in liver enzymes is expected
- Hyperlipidaemia
- Hyperkalaemia
- Anaemia
- Gum hyperplasia
- Convulsions

- Gastric intolerance
- Hypertrichosis
- Immunosuppression

Monitoring

- FBS and ESR
- U&E, creatinine, urate, LFTs
- Fasting lipids, magnesium
- Blood pressure
- Above tests at baseline, at fortnightly intervals for first 3 months, then monthly

Cyclophosphamide

Indications

- RA – particularly with vasculitis, SLE, Wegener's granulomatosis, polyarteritis nodosa

Dose

- Usually given in pulsed IV doses for severe SLE or systemic vasculitis
- Can also be given orally 1mg–1.5 mg/kg daily
- Consider adding oral septrin (sulfamethoxazole/trimethoprim) for *Pneumocystis carinii* prophylaxis

Side Effects

- GIT upset
- Hair loss
- Amenorrhoea/azoospermia – usually reversible on discontinuation of therapy but may cause gonadal failure – consider ovary protection
- Chemical or haemorrhagic cystitis – advise patient about adequate fluid intake (1–2 L/day)
- Pulmonary fibrosis
- Drug interactions
  — allopurinol
  — potentiates effects of sulfonylurea or other hypoglycemic agents

Monitoring

Check FBC and ESR fortnightly for first 8 weeks and then monthly thereafter

Consider Stopping Therapy

If any of the following develops:

- Leucopenia
- Thrombocytopenia
- Severe dysuria
- Significant pulmonary symptoms

Newer Agents in Inflammatory Arthritis

These agents are usually reserved for those with active disease despite MTX or if intolerant of MTX.

Leflunomide

- Inhibits the production of pyrimidine ribonucleotides and hence cell replication
- Loading dose 100 mg daily for 2–3 days, thereafter 10–20 mg daily (loading dose may be omitted – reduces side effects)
- Adverse effects – headache, vomiting, diarrhoea, alopecia, hypertension, marrow toxicity, weight loss
- Men and women should not reproduce while taking leflunomide (teratogenic)
- FBC every 2 weeks for 3 months, LFTs monthly for 6 months
- Extremely long half-life so washout with cholestyramine may be needed for toxicity or unexpected pregnancy

Biological Agents

There has been a dramatic breakthrough in our understanding of the mechanisms of persisting joint inflammation in recent years. Cytokines such as TNF alpha and interleukin 1 have been shown to have a crucial role in maintaining inflammation. Several targeted anti-cytokine therapies have been developed and the agents described below (infliximab, anakinra and etanercept) have been licensed for use in rheumatoid arthritis. They also show great promise for use in other arthropathies, e.g. psoriatic arthritis and ankylosing spondylitis.

These agents are extremely expensive whereas methotrexate, the current first-line therapy for rheumatoid arthritis, is long off patent and is extremely cheap. They are therefore reserved at present for those that methotrexate fails to control.

There has been concern about toxicity of these therapies, especially atypical infection. An excess of cases of tuberculosis reactivation have been reported along with opportunistic infections, e.g. *Pneumocystis carinii* pneumonia. However, a number of large databases of patients on anti-TNF therapy have failed to demonstrate an excess of infection over a 3-year period.

Etanercept

- A recombinant TNF alpha receptor, Fc fusion protein
- Binds to TNF alpha, blocking its interaction with cell surface receptors
- Self administered, 25 mg subcutaneously twice weekly
- Adverse effects – injection site reactions. Rare reports of pancytopenia, aplastic anaemia. Long-term safety unknown; possible ↑ predisposition to malignancy or infection. Some reports of demyelination
- Onset of action in weeks – often given in conjunction with MTX
- chest radiograph and tuberculin test before treatment
- Duration of therapy unknown

Infliximab

- Also anti-TNF alpha. A monoclonal antibody which binds to both serum and membrane bound TNF alpha inhibiting its function
- Administered by IV infusion (3 mg/kg over 2 h) at 0, 2, 6 weeks and thereafter every 8 weeks
- Given in conjunction with MTX
- Adverse effects – acute infusion reactions. Theoretical risk of malignancy and infection as for etanercept. TB reactivation can occur (rarely); chest radiograph and tuberculin test before treatment
- Adequate contraception must be used (as for etanercept)
- Duration of therapy unknown
- Use with extreme caution, if at all in those with significant organ failure (cardiac, renal, hepatic, respiratory)

Anakinra

- Interleukin 1 receptor antagonist (1L-1RA)
- Virtually identical to the naturally occurring form of 1L-1RA
- Daily subcutaneous injection
- Adverse effects – infection site reactions, infections
- Adequate contraception must be used
- Duration of therapy unknown

Joint Injections

Common Indications for Steroid Injection

- Synovitis in one or two joints
- Knee effusion/osteoarthritis
- Soft tissue lesions e.g. rotator cuff, epicondylitis, bursitis

Technique

- Wash hands, wear gloves
- Topical antiseptic (sterile wipes)
- No-touch technique
- Use different needle for drawing up and injecting
- Mark location of injection entry
- Never inject against resistance
- Avoid intradermal injection as it can cause fat necrosis or skin atrophy

Articular Injections

	Wrist	Shoulder	Elbow	Knee	Ankle
Methyl prednisolone	40 mg	40 mg	40 mg	80 mg	40 mg
Trimcinolone acetonide	20 mg	20 mg	20 mg	40 mg	20 mg
(+ 1–4 ml lignocaine/lidocaine to increase volume)					

Injection of small joints (e.g. MCP, PIP, MTP) – methyl prendisolone 20 mg or triamcinolone 10 mg. Methyl prednisolone 20–40 mg for soft tissue injections.

Advice to Patients

- Explain risk of infection (approx. 1:10 000)
- Rarely pain is worse 24 h after injection
- Rest joint for 12–24 h
- Expect relief in 48–72 h

Recurrent Problems

- Repeated injection is not usually the best management – seek advice

How Many Injections is Safe?

- No good data but some rheumatologists wary of more than 3–4 per joint

How Often?

- Little data; most clinicians recommend minimum 3–6 months between injections

Contraindications to Injection

- Bleeding diathesis (but patients on warfarin who are appropriately anticoagulated can usually be injected safely without stopping warfarin)
- Injection near a site of infection
- Joint instability
- Prosthetic joint
- Fracture involving joint

Judicious use of injections for exacerbations of e.g. knee OA in elderly can give benefit for some years where joint surgery not indicated or contraindicated.

Role of Health Professionals

Rheumatology Nurse Specialist (RNS)

The role of the RNS varies between rheumatology departments. Key working areas of the RNS may include:

- Acting as a support for patients. Junior doctors change posts every few months, while the RNS acts as a permanent point of contact within the department
- Acting as a resource for health professionals
  - in the hospital, both within the rheumatology department and in other departments
  - in the community
- Educating patients and their families about their condition and about the risks or benefits of their treatment. Patients commencing a DMARD are referred to the RNS
- Fulfilling the role of a research nurse
- In some departments the RNS has a role in overseeing the monitoring of DMARDs
- The RNS may have a role in assessing patients, similar to the role of the doctor but with greater supervision
- Some nurse specialists administer joint injections e.g. knee, shoulder

Physiotherapist

* Physiotherapy can be useful in the management of musculoskeletal conditions where pain, swelling and loss of range of movement or muscle strength is a problem
* Physiotherapy can help improve patients' mobility and function through a variety of physical means, education and support

Pain and Swelling

Pain can be treated with manual treatment techniques such as mobilisations and manipulations, with exercise and through the use of electrotherapy modalities such as short wave diathermy and ultrasound.

* **Mobilisations** are passive oscillatory movements that are applied to a joint and performed for the purpose of relieving pain and restoring pain-free functional movement
* **Manipulation** is a single high velocity movement of short amplitude, which is not under the control of the patient. It is a treatment technique sometimes performed when no further improvement is possible with mobilisation
* **Heat** is used to treat pain and reduce swelling and may be applied in different ways. The method of heating by conduction as in wax treatment, hot packs and hydrotherapy has a superficial effect on tissues. High frequency currents such as short wave diathermy and ultrasound penetrate deeper lying structures
* **Short wave diathermy** produces an electromagnetic field to generate heat
* **Ultrasound** is high frequency sound waves, which cause tissue cells to oscillate in the ultrasonic beam. Ultrasound is claimed to reduce oedema and soften scar tissue
* **Interferential therapy** is a medium frequency electrical treatment, used for pain reduction
* There is a paucity of controlled data demonstrating benefits of heat and electrotherapy

Flexibility

Chronically shortened tissues (from occupational or postural stress) can be stretched using manual soft tissue stretching techniques and massage to increase muscle and connective tissue length and flexibility.

Range of Movement

Joint range of movement can be increased with mobilisation treatment, traction and exercise. Traction can be either manual or mechanical

Muscle Strength

Muscles can be strengthened both regionally and segmentally through exercise training for the purposes of improving physical endurance and conditioning.

Muscles that are weak or atrophied can be electrically stimulated using a neuromuscular electrical stimulator. This delivers low frequency electrical impulses to improve tone and muscle strength.

Mobility and Function

Physiotherapists have much to offer in areas such as improving balance and confidence in walking. They also offer advice where appropriate on posture and injury prevention. Some specialise in the provision of orthotic devices.

Some physiotherapists have begun to adopt complementary therapies such as acupuncture and acupressure.

Occupational Therapist

The OT has a distinct role, but some aspects overlap with the physiotherapist and nurse specialist.

- Joint protection education – makes intuitive sense but has not been proven to "protect" joints from damage or deformity
- Provision of splints – usage less common since use of e.g. IM Methylprednisolone for flares of RA. Compliance with medium–long-term use is poor. Knee brace for joint instability can be highly effective
- Provision of assistive devices – useful for the relatively small percentage of patients with more severe disability
- House modification – again, may be essential for those with more severe disability
- Energy conservation/relaxation – role overlaps with physiotherapist/ nurse specialist
- Vocational Retraining – usually not undertaken by rheumatology departments

Soft Tissue Problems 9

Fibromyalgia Syndrome (FMS)

- Accounts for up to 20% of new rheumatology referrals
- Appears to be primarily a manifestation of chronic psychosocial distress, which results in abnormal sensory processing in the CNS
- Is a diagnosis of exclusion characterised by poor sleep pattern, global muscle pain, fatigability and irritability. Associated with irritable bowel syndrome, tension headaches, chronic fatigue syndrome
- Often co-exists with diseases such as SLE and RA (prevalence of FMS in those with SLE is 30% and causes most of the musculoskeletal pain)

History

- Diffuse muscle pain for 3 months minimum
- Psychological factors – "stress", anxiety/tension, difficulty relaxing, depressive features
- Fatigue, poor sleep

Examination

- Multiple tender muscle sites (but not everyone with FMS will be tender at all sites):
  — lower cervical spine
  — midpoint supraspinatus
  — trapezius
  — 1 cm distal to lateral epicondyle
  — lower lumbar spine
  — upper gluteal region
  — pectoralis
  — medial fat pad of knee
- Articular exam normal

Investigation

- ESR, CPK normal and RF and ANA negative. Consider thyroid function tests
- A number of papers have documented increased substance P in the CSF in FMS, significance uncertain

Management

- Make the diagnosis. Patients control their symptoms better when they have a diagnosis
- Empathise. This pain is real. Have you ever had abdominal cramps or diarrhoea before an examination or interview? That was due to acute "stress". FMS is associated with chronic "stress"
- Emphasise self-help through reassurance and education. Try to reduce/eliminate stressors
- Refer to OT/RNS/physiotherapist, as appropriate, for assistance with the above
- Self-help group for fibromyalgia patients where available
- Encourage aerobic exercise. Many with fibromyalgia don't exercise as it worsens pain. Reassure that exercise will not worsen their condition or cause damage. Gradually increase exercise. Forms of exercise with a social component (e.g. aerobics or dance classes) are more likely to be continued than solitary exercise
- Address psychological distress, underlying anxiety, depression
- Amitriptyline 25 mg at night if sleep disturbed

Neck Pain/Low Back Pain

A very common symptom, but:

- Prevalence of disease e.g. disc protrusion, ankylosing spondylitis, spondylolisthesis, bony secondaries, is low in both acute and chronic pain. The presence of normal age related spondylotic changes on radiographs, e.g. osteophyte formation, disc space narrowing, in those >40 years correlates poorly with neck and low back pain
- **Acute pain** associated with muscle spasm and reduced movement common. Responds to analgesics, muscle relaxants, physiotherapy interventions. Observational evidence for response to chiropractic manipulation. Relatively little controlled/comparative data. Continue normal activities as far as possible
- **Chronic pain** (more than 8–12 weeks) is in general a complex problem and needs to be treated as such. One study (*NEJM* 1999; 340(5): 389–90) showed no overall difference between chiropractic manipulation, physiotherapy or reading an information booklet only in chronic low back pain. Rare cases of spinal cord or brain injury have been reported with manipulation. Prolonged bed rest is contraindicated. Those who do best remain mobile and continue usual activities as far as possible

If pain persists for more than 6 weeks, consider if psychosocial factors are contributing. Psychosocial distress, a very common problem, is frequently associated with neck or low back pain. When associated with tender muscles in a particular distribution = FMS. Psychological factors also affect the progression of acute to chronic pain, e.g. lack of job satisfaction is a strong predictor of the development of chronic pain in those with acute pain.

Management of Chronic Neck/Low Back Pain

As for FMS:

- Good management leading to pain reduction and improved function requires considerable skill (stronger analgesics usually not the answer)
- Avoid overinvestigation (but see "Red Flags" section)
- Reassure about absence of evidence of disease
- Acknowledge reality of pain felt. Ask whether stress/frustration could be part of the overall clinical picture
- Encourage robust attitude but remain empathic
- Reassure that normal activities may cause pain but will not worsen the condition (where no disease found)
- Refer to physiotherapist, occupational therapist, as appropriate, and subsequently hand control of symptoms back to the patient
- Occasional referral to psychologist, pain clinic

Pain Clinics

Those with chronic musculoskeletal pain may benefit, in certain circumstances, from assessment at a pain clinic. Staffed commonly by anaesthetists, psychologists and other professionals they offer a range of physical (e.g. transcutaneous nerve stimulation, nerve blockade, facet joint injection, epidural) or psychological (e.g. cognitive behavioural therapy) interventions. Discuss with rheumatologist if referral considered. Some rheumatologists perform epidurals themselves.

Red Flags in Spinal Pain

Further investigation and definitive diagnosis required if:
- Age <20, >55
- Prolonged stiffness, energy ↓, weight loss, unwell
- Thoracic pain
- Night time pain
- Abnormal neurological signs
- History of TB /cancer /steroid use
- ↑ ESR, abnormal FBC or bone profile, ↑ prostate specific antigen

Practice Point

Full history and general examination is important in all presenting with back pain, e.g. aortic aneurysm, endometriosis, metastatic malignancy can all present with low back pain.

Disc Protrusion

- Often acute onset; worse with coughing, sneezing
- Neck or low back pain with unilateral radiation in distribution of affected nerve root
- Associated paraesthesiae and muscle weakness as per affected nerve root (see table – Sign and Symptoms of Common Disc Lesions)
- Stretching affected nerve causes pain in distribution of nerve, e.g. sciatic stretch test, femoral nerve stretch test
- Presence of urinary or bowel symptoms (altered perianal sensation, difficulty voiding, loss of control) = cauda equina syndrome, a medical emergency that needs urgent neurosurgical assessment

Investigation

- CT or MRI (lumbar), MRI (cervical) usually performed when surgery contemplated or where diagnosis uncertain
- Considerable radiation dose from CT. Routine CT lumbar spine scans only lower 3 lumbar disc levels ($L_{3/4}$–L_5S_1) so you must specifically request more levels if indicated

Management

- Acute – analgesics, muscle relaxants, balance rest/activity, as above
- Epidural injection of long-acting anaesthetic and steroid useful in some circumstances
- Most disc protrusions settle spontaneously in days to weeks
- Surgery occasionally indicated (discectomy) for severe symptoms or neurological compromise

Practice Point

Prevalence of asymptomatic disc bulge, disc protrusion or nerve root compression on MRI is up to 10% of normal population. It is therefore important to correlate symptoms, signs and imaging abnormalities, especially when surgery is considered.

Signs and Symptoms of Common Disc Lesions

Disc	Root	Distribution of pain	Motor	Sensory	Reflex
Cervical					
$C_{5/6}$	C_6	Shoulder/Lateral arm	Biceps, Wrist extension	Thumb/Index finger	Biceps
$C_{6/7}$	C_7	Shoulder/Lateral arm	Triceps, Finger extension, Wrist flex	Index/Middle finger	Triceps
C_7/T_1	C_8	Medial arm/Forearm	Finger flex, Intrinsic muscles	Ring and little fingers	Triceps
Lumbar					
$L_{3/4}$	L_4	Anterolateral thigh, Medial knee	Knee extension	Anterolateral thigh	Quadriceps
$L_{4/5}$	L_5	Posterior thigh/ Lateral calf, Dorsum of foot	Ankle dorsiflexion, Extension great toe	Posterolateral calf, Dorsum of foot	No specific reflex
L_5/S_1	S_1	Buttock, Post Thigh, Calf, Foot, Lateral toes	Ankle plantar flexion	As for pain distribution	Achilles

The above signs may be present to varying degrees with disc protrusions.

Spinal Stenosis

- Narrowing of lumbar spinal canal. Usually degenerative due to combination of facet joint osteoarthritis and ligamentum flavum hypertrophy. Congenital narrowing may contribute
- Age 60+

- Low back/buttock pain, radiates to legs. Predominately or exclusively exertional. Similar to vascular claudication (called neurogenic claudication)

Investigation
- CT scan demonstrates bone overgrowth, ligamentous hypertrophy ± congenital narrowing

Management
- Physiotherapy, facet injection, epidural effective in some
- Surgical decompression if symptoms severe or interfering with function

Scheuermann's Disease
- Vertebral osteochondritis occurring in adolescence. Most commonly affects thoracic vertebrae
- Often asymptomatic. Can be associated with spinal pain particularly if lumbar spine involved. Painless dorsal kyphosis in adulthood is often secondary to Scheuermann's disease
- Radiographs show irregularity of vertebral end plates, anterior vertebral wedging, and kyphosis

Whiplash Injury
Sudden, violent, unexpected, flexion and extension of the neck. If severe can cause cord injury and death. Most injuries are relatively minor but are difficult to judge clinically and radiographically (including MRI). Speed of impact and amount of damage to vehicle correlate to a degree with severity of injury. At least 80% get better over 6 months. Remainder can have a constellation of symptoms lasting months to years (late whiplash syndrome). Prevalence low in countries with no monetary compensation systems.
Three factors account for persistence of symptoms:

- Unrecognised or severe injury
  — blocking nerves to facet joints in chronic whiplash when compared to sham blockade has been shown (*NEJM* 1996; 335(23): 1721–6) to improve symptoms considerably
- Psychosocial factors
  — as for chronic neck/low back pain
  — presence of injury through no fault of their own, prospect of a court case adds to "stress".
  — some develop features of fibromyalgia
- Malingering
  — a factor in some cases but not in a majority.

Management
- As for chronic neck/low back pain. Advise patients to settle any legal actions sooner rather than waiting for symptoms to resolve

Shoulder Pain

Common Problems

- Rotator cuff disorders, especially tendonitis
- Adhesive capsulitis
- Biceps tendonitis

Osteoarthritis of the shoulder joint is uncommon, apart from Acromio-clavicular (AC) joint OA. Arthritis of the shoulder (i.e. glenohumeral joint) is usually part of an oligo- or polyarticular inflammatory arthropathy.

Rotator Cuff Muscles (Mnemonic SITS)

S supraspinatus
I infraspinatus
T teres minor
S subscapularis

History

- Pain originating in the shoulder is usually felt over deltoid and the upper arm
- Pain over trapezius or over scapula is most often cervical in origin (exception: AC joint)

The affected shoulder is usually sore to lie on, and pure shoulder movements, e.g. reaching into cupboard or behind back, are painful

Examination

- Inspection – muscle wasting (especially posteriorly), swelling, deformity. Inspection of shoulder may appear normal, even in severe disease
- Palpation – tenderness (often non specific), swelling, joint instability
- Movement – assess active and passive movement in abduction, adduction, flexion, extension, internal/external rotation

Rotator Cuff Disorders

- Cause pain and may result in some limitation of active movements but passive movements are usually preserved
- Pain is felt especially on resisted movement, particularly abduction
- Painful arc of abduction 80–110° with supraspinatus impingement.

Adhesive Capsulitis

- Causes pain on active and passive movements; there is global reduction of all movements with a "doughy" feel at the end of the range of movement

Investigation

- Plain radiographs – if diagnosis uncertain
- Consider MRI – if rotator cuff tear suspected, e.g. loss of active abduction and weakness of abduction and external rotation
- Severe pain, not responding to physiotherapy, injection

Treatment

- Rest
- Analgesics/NSAIDs
- Physiotherapy
- Steroid injection – subacromial (tendonitis), or intra-articular (capsulitis)
- Oral steroid – very occasionally for capsulitis
- Suprascapular nerve block
- Surgical referral – for rotator cuff tear or resistant tendonitis

Carpal Tunnel Syndrome

- An entrapment neuropathy. Occurs when the median nerve is compressed under the flexor retinaculum at the wrist
- Mostly idiopathic. Consider weight gain, pregnancy, myxoedema, trauma, fluid retention, inflammatory arthritis

Symptoms

- Paraesthesiae and pain in radial three fingers and half of the ring finger. Usually worse at night. Pain may be felt above the wrist

Signs

- Tinel's sign and Phalen's sign have relatively poor sensitivity and specificity
- Altered sensation in median nerve distribution
- Weakness of thumb abduction/thenar wasting in advanced cases
- Consider cervical origin if symptoms atypical

Investigations

- Nerve conduction studies (especially if motor abnormality present or doubt about diagnosis)

Treatment

- NSAIDs
- Splinting
- Local corticosteroid injection
- Surgical release of transverse carpal ligament
- Indications for surgery:
  - inadequate response to injection
  - muscle weakness or atrophy

Epicondylitis

Lateral Epicondylitis (Tennis Elbow)

- Enthesitis – "inflammation" of common extensor origin at lateral epicondyle of humerus

Diagnosis

- Pain over lateral aspect of elbow, worse with activity such as lifting a cup
- Tenderness of the lateral epicondyle **and**
- Pain felt at the lateral epicondyle on resisted extension of the wrist

Management

- Rest
- NSAIDs
- Local corticosteroid injection

Medial Epicondylitis (Golfer's Elbow)

- Inflammation of common flexor origin at the medial epicondyle

Diagnosis

- Pain over medial aspect of elbow, worse on lifting with a flexed wrist
- Tender medial epicondyle **and**
- Pain felt on medial side of elbow on resisted wrist flexion or pronation

Management

- As for tennis elbow

Bursitis

A bursa is a sac with a potential space that facilitates one tissue in gliding over another.

Common Sites of Bursitis

Trochanteric Bursitis

- Pain felt over lateral aspect of hip especially over greater trochanter
- Pain can be exacerbated by lying on the affected side, walking and external rotation of the hip
- Some have lower limb mechanical problem e.g. short leg, knee or ankle abnormality

Prepatellar Bursitis

- Pain, swelling and warmth over the prepatellar bursa, located superficial to the patella
- Caused by repetitive trauma or overuse, e.g. kneeling

Olecranon Bursitis (Student's Elbow)

- Pain, swelling and warmth over the olecranon process
- Elbow usually has normal range of movement unless the bursa is extremely tense with fluid

Subacromial Bursitis

- Pain on active shoulder movement, especially abduction, with much less pain or no pain on passive movements. May be difficult to distinguish from rotator cuff tendonitis

Treatment

- If bursa is large and fluid filled, can aspirate
- Gram stain, culture and sensitivity, when appropriate, to rule out infection. Look for crystals (gout, pseudogout, cholesterol as a potential cause)
- If infection ruled out, inject with corticosteroid

De Quervain's Tenosynovitis

- Inflammation of sheath of abductor pollicis and extensor pollicis brevis
- Pain felt at radial side of wrist, proximal to 1st CMC joint

Examination

- Tenderness along line of tendons at or just proximal to anatomical snuffbox with some local swelling
- Positive Finklestein's test:
  Ask patient to make a fist over their flexed thumb, then passively move the wrist in ulnar deviation → pain = positive test

Treatment

- Inject tendon sheath
- Occasionally splint
- Physiotherapy

Achilles Tendonitis

- Inflammation of Achilles tendon
- Often a misuse or overuse injury
- Occasionally due to seronegative spondylarthropathy

Examination

- Soft tissue swelling over tendon with local tenderness
- May be difficult to distinguish, without ultrasound, from Achilles bursitis
- Feel for a "dip" in Achilles, raising possibility of a tear
- Ultrasound scan if any uncertainty

Treatment

- Rest
- Physiotherapy
- Careful peritendinous injection with hydrocortisone can be very effective (do not attempt this yourself). Ideally should be performed under ultrasound guidance
- Some rheumatologists do not inject because of risk of tendon rupture

Plantar Fasciitis

- Inflammation of plantar fascia insertion into calcaneus
- A typical feature of seronegative spondylarthropathies
- Most heel pain is not due to plantar fasciitis but originates in the heel pad (fat pad syndrome). The two conditions may be difficult to distinguish as tenderness over middle of the heel pad is seen in both
- Finding a calcaneal spur on a radiograph does not correlate with heel pain – only useful to look for erosion or periostitis of plantar fasciitis secondary to spondylarthropathy

Treatment

- Heel cup inserted into shoe
- May require valgus support if fixed or passively correctable hind foot deformity also present
- Occasionally steroid injection required but avoid repeat injection – can cause heel pad atrophy and worsen the condition

Benign Hypermobility Syndrome

- A syndrome characterised by varying degrees of joint laxity without instability or disability
- Has a familial tendency. Most commonly affects young women
- Arthralgia (most commonly of hands, knees and hips) occurs with unusual physical activity and frequent wrist or ankle sprains can occur
- At least three of the six tests for hypermobility are needed to make the diagnosis

Six Tests for Joint Hypermobility

1 Passive abduction of the thumb to touch flexor surface of the forearm
2 Passive extension of the MCP joints to 90°
3 >10° hyperextension at the elbow
4 >10° hyperextension at the knee (genu recurvatum)
5 Trunk flexion so that the palms of the hands can be placed flat on the ground
6 Dorsiflexion of the ankle 20° past a right angle

Differential Diagnosis of Joint Hypermobility

- Benign hypermobility (most common)
- Ehlers–Danlos syndrome
- Marfan's syndrome
- Osteogenesis imperfecta

All are associated with defects in type I collagen. Joint hypermobility and skin hyperextensibility are seen to varying degrees in all of the above.

Ehlers–Danlos Syndrome (EDS)

Clinical Features

- Velvety, soft skin
- Hyperextensible skin and joints
- Cigarette paper scars
- Easy bruising
- Scoliosis
- Osteoporosis
- Aneurysm

Diagnosis

- Clinical pattern
- Skin biopsy – fibroblast analysis in order to determine type of EDS and therefore risk of complications

Marfan's Syndrome

- Tall, thin
- Upper/lower body ratio 0.85 (normal = 0.93)
- Arm span > height > 1.05
- Arachnodactyly
  - thumb sign – thumb protrudes beyond ulnar border of palm when patient makes a fist over the thumb
  - wrist signs – thumb and little finger overlap on circling the opposite wrist
- Upward dislocation of lens (need a slit lamp to see)
- Aortic root dilation in 50% of children. Check annually in adults
- Beta-blocker reduces risk of aortic dissection in pregnancy

Osteogenesis Imperfecta (OGI)

- Abnormal bone matrix with secondary osteoporosis
- Scleral hue (type I)
- Dentinogenesis imperfecta
- Scoliosis
- Joint laxity
- Easy bruising
- Hearing loss

Osteoarthritis 10

- Common chronic joint condition. Primarily a disease of cartilage
- Increasing evidence of inflammation in early osteoarthritis
- The clinical hallmark is **bony swelling** of the affected joint
- Distinct pattern of joint involvement in primary OA:
  - distal interphalangeal joints (Heberden's nodes)
  - PIP joints (Bouchard's)
  - 1st carpometacarpal joint (CMC) – thumb base pain – pain taking lids off jars, turning on taps
  - acromioclavicular joint (AC) – tip of shoulder pain
  - hip – pain in groin and anteromedial thigh
  - knee (patello-femoral and tibio-femoral)
  - 1st metatarsophalangeal joint (MTP)
- Secondary OA can occur at site of previous trauma or inflammation. Therefore OA affecting unusual sites e.g. MCP, wrist, elbow, gleno-humeral joint, ankle – may need investigation to rule out secondary causes, e.g. pyrophosphate arthropathy
- Cervical and lumbar spondylosis = OA of spine – affects facet joints predominantly. Associated vertebral osteophytes and disc space narrowing

Investigations

- Bloods – normal
- Radiographs:
  - loss of joint space
  - subchondral sclerosis
  - peripheral osteophytes
  - subchondral cysts
  - deformity

Treatment (in order)

- Patient education/reassurance
- Exercises to improve muscle strength, e.g. gluteal for hip, quadriceps for knee OA
- Analgesic options
  - NSAIDs for short term or occasional use
  - analgesics – paracetamol, solpadeine, codeine preparations
  - topical capsaicin, anti-inflammatory gels
- Joint aspiration and steroid injection – judicious use of injection for exacerbations of, e.g. knee OA, can give benefit for some years where surgery not indicated or contraindicated
- Hyaluronic acid injection – multiple injections required over a short period (approximately 3 weeks). Consistent data demonstrating efficacy is lacking
- Walking stick
  - hip OA – hold stick in contralateral hand
  - knee OA – hold stick in ipsilateral hand
- Surgery
  - severe disease with decreased mobility
  - night pain
  - joint instability

Diffuse Idiopathic Skeletal Hyperostosis (DISH)

- Usually seen in patients >50 years
- Spinal stiffness common, but patients may be asymptomatic. Spinal range of movement reduced
- Plain radiographs demonstrate bone proliferation at vertebral margins and ligamentous ossification
- Preservation of disc spaces and normal facet joints differentiate it from osteoarthritis
- Normal sacroiliac joints help distinguish DISH from ankylosing spondylitis
- More common in diabetes mellitus
- Management is symptomatic

Rheumatoid Arthritis 11

Rheumatoid arthritis (RA) is the classic example of a chronic inflammatory arthritis. Chronic joint inflammation, whatever the cause, can damage joints permanently within a few months (MRI can demonstrate irrevocable joint damage in RA within **weeks** of onset). DMARDs can prevent or reduce this damage, especially when started early. It is therefore very important to learn to recognise joint inflammation (synovitis) so that appropriate treatment can be given. The signs of joint inflammation may be subtle and the assessment of disease activity is not an all-or-nothing decision, but is based on a composite of the following variables:

- Duration and severity of morning stiffness (>1 hour suggests activity)
- Number of swollen joints
- Number of tender joints
- Lab. variables, e.g.
  - acute phase reactants – ESR$\uparrow$, CRP$\uparrow$, serum amyloid A $\uparrow$
  - haemoglobin ($\downarrow$)
  - platelet count ($\uparrow$)

The aim of the rheumatologist is to suppress inflammation as completely and as quickly as possible. When there are signs of inflammation, e.g. swollen/tender joint or elevated ESR and diseases causing bone erosion (e.g. RA, spondylarthropathy) enter the differential diagnosis, the patient needs to be reviewed by a rheumatologist.

NSAIDs alone are **not** adequate therapy for inflammation lasting any more than 1–2 weeks associated with these diseases.

Differential Diagnosis of Inflammatory Arthritis

- **Rheumatoid arthritis**
- **Sero-negative spondylarthropathy**
  - ankylosing spondylitis
  - psoriatic arthropathy
  - reactive arthritis
  - enteropathic arthritis
  - Behçet's disease
- **Connective tissue disease**
  - SLE
  - scleroderma
  - Sjögren's syndrome
  - polymyositis, dermatomyositis
  - mixed connective tissue disease
- **Crystal arthritis**
  - gout
  - pseudogout
- **Arthritis associated with infection**
  - bacterial
  - viral
  - fungal (rare)
  - spirochaete (*Borrelia burgdorferi*, Lyme disease)
- **Vasculitis**
  - e.g. Wegener's granulomatosis, polyarteritis nodosa, giant cell arteritis
- **Sarcoidosis**
  - periarthritis
- **Polymyalgia rheumatica**
  - Evidence of joint effusion ± small joint synovitis

Rheumatoid Arthritis

- Symmetrical inflammatory polyarthropathy that affects females with a 3 : 1 predominance. Prevalence 0.2–0.5% of population
- Onset may be abrupt or insidious
- Incidence may be declining. Mean age of onset is 48 years
- Affects particularly:
  — hands – MCPs and PIPs
  — wrists
  — elbows, shoulders, neck
  — knees, ankles and subtalar joints
  — feet – midtarsal and MTP joints
  — temporomandibular joint
- Spares DIP joints, thoracolumbar spine

American College of Rheumatology Classification Criteria

For classification as RA, any four of the following criteria must be met and be present for at least 6 weeks (note that these are not diagnostic criteria):

1. Morning stiffness in and around joints lasting at least 1 hour before maximal improvement
2. Soft tissue swelling (synovitis) of three or more joints
3. Synovitis of PIP, MCP or wrist joints
4. Symmetrical arthropathy
5. Subcutaneous nodules
6. Positive test for rheumatoid factor
7. Radiographic erosions or periarticular osteopenia in hand or wrist joints

Mnemonic "EARS"

- **E**arly morning stiffness
- **A**rthritis ≥ 3 joints, hands involved
- **R**heumatoid factor, rheumatoid nodules, radiological changes
- **S**ymmetrical arthritis

Examination

- Assess number of tender and swollen joints
- Look and palpate for tenosynovitis in hands and feet
- Look for mechanical problems:
  — loss of power, especially grip
  — loss of range of movement
  — check stability of joints, e.g. elbow/knee

- In long established disease look for evidence of upper motor neurone signs in limbs secondary to cervical cord compression, e.g. hyperreflexia, clonus, extensor plantar
- Look for signs of extraskeletal disease: (usually in long established disease), e.g.:
  — splinter haemorrhages, nail fold infarcts (1–2 mm black/brown lesions at the nail folds, a sign of small-vessel vasculitis)
  — rheumatoid nodules
  — sicca syndrome
  — median nerve entrapment
  — proteinuria (raising possibility of amyloidosis).
- Uncommon features need not be sought at each visit, e.g. pulmonary fibrosis, pericarditis, splenomegaly (+ neutropenia = Felty's syndrome), episcleritis, scleromalacia

Practice Point

Inflamed rheumatoid joints do not go red. Suspect sepsis in a rheumatoid patient with a red joint.

Investigations

- FBC
- Normochromic normocytic anaemia
- Increased platelets with active disease
- Occasional leucopenia – Felty's syndrome
- Pancytopenia – rare, usually drug induced
- ↑ alkaline phosphatase with active disease
- ESR – useful indicator of disease activity
- CRP – more sensitive than ESR
- Rheumatoid factor
  — positive in 70% of patients with RA
  — the higher the titre, the greater the significance but it is not diagnostic in itself. RF titre does not reflect disease activity
  — no need to remeasure in those already seropositive
- Antinuclear antibody – positive in 50–70% of patients with RA
- Radiography:
  — chest radiograph– if commencing on methotrexate or has symptoms of pulmonary disease
  — hands and feet – to assess for joint erosions
  — other radiographic features
    — periarticular osteoporosis
    — joint space loss
    — soft tissue swelling
    — deformity
  — X-ray joints that appear deformed or damaged but not inflamed joints. Discuss with rheumatologist or speciality trainee

- consider need for DEXA as bone mineral density frequently low in RA
- In long standing RA X-ray cervical spine (lateral view in flexion and extension) for evidence of atlantoaxial subluxation
- Joint aspiration – examine for white cell count and differential, and culture and sensitivity if any suspicion of sepsis

Treatment

- It is important to treat early and aggressively, to prevent long-term deformity and disability
- Mainstay of treatment is a DMARD and low dose corticosteroids. The latter is not universally accepted as some rheumatologists feel the risks outweigh the benefits. The benefits are:
  - symptomatic
  - evidence for reduction in frequency and severity of bone erosion with low dose oral steroids

DMARDs

- Methotrexate, sulfasalazine, hydroxychloroquine, leflunomide, infliximab, etanercept, anakinra, cyclosporin – see relevant pages for dosage, monitoring, side effects, etc
- Gold, penicillamine, azathioprine – less commonly used now

Corticosteroids

- IM methylprednisolone 120 mg for very active disease
- IV methylprednisolone 500 mg for severe active disease (rarely)
- Oral dose of 5–7.5 mg daily maintenance therapy, wean if disease control good, add bone prophylaxis (see osteoporosis)
- Maintenance doses >7.5 mg to be avoided
- Judicious steroid injection of individual joints and/or tendon sheaths

NSAIDs

Non-drug Treatment

- Physiotherapy
- Occupational therapy
- RNS referral
- Podiatry and chiropody (including custom-made shoes)
- Consider orthopaedic opinion for damaged joints or for prevention e.g. of tendon rupture (discuss with rheumatologist). Among the more common surgical interventions are carpal tunnel decompression, removal of ulnar styloid (prevention of extensor digiti minimi rupture), knee and hip arthroplasty. Ankle arthrodesis and metatarsal head excision can be very effective for pain reduction. Stabilisation of cervical spine subluxation, elbow and shoulder surgery also occasionally required

Seronegative Spondylarthropathy

12

A group of five heterogeneous diseases (psoriatic arthropathy, ankylosing spondylitis, reactive arthritis, enteropathic arthritis, and Behçet's disease) linked together by a number of articular, extra-articular and genetic features. Seronegative rheumatoid arthritis is not part of the group.

Occasionally, patients present with features of spondylarthropathy (e.g. knee arthropathy, Achilles tendonitis and sacro-iliitis) but do not fit into any one of the five diseases. This is classified as undifferentiated spondylarthropathy.

Associated Features

All of the features are not seen in each disease and vary in their prevalence (0–100%).

- Asymmetrical oligoarthritis/occasionally monoarthritis
- Presence of enthesitis, i.e. inflammation at origin or insertion of ligament or tendon into bone, e.g. Achilles tendonitis, plantar fasciitis
- High prevalence of HLA B27
- Involvement of sacroiliac joints, either uni- or bilateral
- Spinal inflammation, i.e. spondylitis
- Extra-articular features e.g. iritis, aortic regurgitation

Treatment

- Sulfasalazine or methotrexate is used for persisting peripheral joint inflammation
- Methotrexate effect on spinal inflammation debateable but may be effective
- Anti-TNF agents appear very effective for both peripheral joint and axial joint inflammation

Psoriatic Arthritis

- Occurs in approximately 7% of those with psoriasis
- Various clinical patterns are recognised:
  - DIP joint involvement with nail changes
  - symmetrical (like RA)
  - arthritis mutilans with digit destruction
  - ankylosing spondylitis pattern
  - asymmetrical disease affecting hands and feet

Clinical Features

- Skin lesions usually precede arthritis
- Skin involvement may be minimal, e.g. dry scalp or natal cleft only even when joint involvement significant
- Nail changes include pitting, onycholysis and thickening/ discoloration
- Occasionally nail changes only present
- Dactylitis a feature: swelling of a digit, either finger or toe, often associated with redness of overlying skin is due to the combination of synovitis and tenosynovitis.

Investigation

- Bloods – FBC, Hb ↓, ESR ↑ (but may be normal despite active disease), RF negative
- Radiography:
  - asymmetrical disease, including sacro-iliac joints; bone erosion and periostitis
  - DIP joint involvement and little or no periarticular osteoporosis
  - syndesmophytes in spine

Treatment

- Sulfasalazine 1 g twice daily
- Joint injection as appropriate
- Methotrexate in severe disease
- NSAIDs – in conjunction with sulfasalazine if needed
- Dermatology referral if psoriasis difficult to control

Ankylosing Spondylitis

- A chronic inflammatory disorder typically affecting the spine and sacroiliac joints (SIJ), which may lead to ossification of ligaments

- Much of the spinal pathology seen in AS is due to enthesopathy
- Fairly common – about 1 : 200 men but less often affects women
- Onset late teens to 20s

History

- Prominent spinal stiffness, night time pain
- Reduced neck and back movement
- Peripheral joint involvement
- Eye involvement
- Interference with activities of daily living

Examination

- Evidence of spinal involvement: reduction of cervical spine, thoracic spine and lumbar spine movement. Reduced chest expansion. Occiput to wall distance in cm, finger floor distance anteriorly and laterally to R+L are often used to assess improvement or deterioration
- Protruberant abdomen
- Enthesitis, e.g. lateral epicondyle, Achilles tendon, plantar fascia
- SIJ involvement – very difficult to assess SIJs clinically
- Peripheral joints – hips and shoulders most commonly
- Other systems
  - CVS – aortic regurgitation
  - RS – upper lobe fibrosis
  - eyes – uveitis
  - skin – psoriatic lesions/nail disease
  - CNS – myelopathy

Investigation

- Bloods
  - FBC, HB↓, platelets ↑ with active disease
  - ESR ↑ in active disease (but doesn't always correlate)
  - LFTs
  - HLA B27 occasionally useful where diagnosis uncertain but prevalence of B27 high in normal population. Finding B27 positive increases possibility of spondylarthropathy but does not make the diagnosis
- Radiography:
  - spine
    - marginal syndesmophytes (vertical calcification of annulus fibres of intervertebral discs)
    - spinal ligament calcification
    - apophyseal joint fusion

    — SIJ
        — bilateral sacroiliitis
        — ↑ uptake in SIJs on isotope bone scan can be unreliable in young adults
        — CT SIJ or gadolinium enhanced MRI useful to look for erosions or signs of inflammation where diagnosis uncertain
    — ± chest radiograph
- Consider
    — ECG
    — PFTs

Treatment

- Sulfasalazine for peripheral joint involvement
- Active exercise to prevent stiffness and deformity. Importance of exercise to preserve spinal movement strongly emphasised although compliance with daily exercise is often poor
- NSAIDs
- Peripheral joint injection
- Occasionally methotrexate
- Anti-TNF agents very effective, likely to be increasingly used, even in relatively early disease

Reactive Arthritis (ReA)

- Acute inflammatory oligoarthritis developing days to weeks after infection
- Typically occurs in 3rd–4th decade
- Source of infection usually gastrointestinal (*Salmonella, Yersinia* most common, also *Shigella, Campylobacter*) or genitourinary (*Chlamydia, Ureaplasma*). May be respiratory in origin
- Is not a septic arthritis, i.e. organisms are not isolated from affected joints. Bacterial antigens have been found in affected joints
- High prevalence of HLA B27 in ReA
- Arthropathy usually lower limb, asymmetrical, dactylitis a feature Sacroiliitis and spinal inflammation also occur
- Extra-articular:
    — Circinate balanitis – inflammation of the glans penis (usually painless)
    — keratoderma blenorrhagica – hyperkerototic psoriasis-like lesions on soles and palms
- Reiter's syndrome – triad of reactive arthritis, conjunctivitis, urethritis occasionally seen. Many develop reactive arthritis without clinical eye or genitourinary involvement

- Presence of urethritis does not necessarily imply genitourinary infection, as urinary tract inflammation can be a feature of reactive arthritis, e.g. gastrointestinal source of infection can result in urethritis

Investigations

- ESR ↑
- Radiograph of SIJs may demonstrate asymmetric sacroiliitis (<50%)
- Stool culture
- Throat swab
- Urethral swab – GU referral if suspect ReA and GI history negative
- Serology for *Salmonella, Yersinia, Chlamydia* where available

Management

- NSAID
- Joint injection
- Oral steroids occasionally
- Treat precipitating infection (does not appear to influence synovitis)
- Sulfasalazine or methotrexate for persisting synovitis
- Approximately 20% develop chronic peripheral or axial arthritis

Arthritis Associated with Inflammatory Bowel Disease (IBD)

- Seen in ulcerative colitis (UC) and Crohn's disease
- Prevalence 2–20% of patients with IBD
- May affect peripheral joints, sacroiliac joints and spine
- Peripheral joint movement usually lower limb, oligoarticular and asymmetrical (typically knee, ankle or MTP and non-erosive)
- Enthesopathy may occur
- Flare of UC is associated with flare of peripheral joint arthritis but spinal symptoms are independent of GI disease activity
- HLA B27 positive in 40–60% with spinal or sacroiliac involvement but is not associated with peripheral arthritis

Management

- NSAIDS
- Joint injection
- Sulfasalazine, occasionally methotrexate

Behçet's Disease

Uncommon in Northern Europe. Often included with the spondyl-arthropathies because the arthritis may involve the spine. Also Behçet's shares many common features with Crohn's disease. However, sacroilitis, HLA B27 and enthesitis are not features of Behçet's disease.

1 Mucosal → oral ulcers (100% of patients)
2 Cutaneous → genital ulcers
3 Skin ulcers/erythema nodosum
4 Uveal → iritis
5 Positive pathergy test → 2 mm erythema 24 h after # 25G needle-prick to depth of 5 mm

Classification Criteria

Need 1 plus two of 2, 3, 4, 5 to satisfy criteria.

Other Features

- Mono/oligoarthritis
- Intestinal ulcers
- Venous/arterial thrombosis
- Meningoencephalitis/cranial nerve palsies

Tests

- HLA B5 is more frequent than HLA B27
- Pathergy reaction
- ESR ↑
- FBC → NN anaemia
- Ophthalmology/dermatology review

Treatment

- NSAIDs
- Treat complications
- Methotrexate/azathioprine/cyclosporin for severe inflammation, e.g. ocular, intestinal
- Iritis → topical or oral steroids
- Mouth ulcers
  — adcortyl in orabase
  — occasionally colchicine
  — dapsone/thalidomide (rarely used)
  — anti-TNF agents reported to be effective

Connective Tissue Diseases (CTD) **13**

Five diseases:

- Systemic lupus erythematosus (SLE)
- Scleroderma
- Polymyositis/dermatomyositis
- Sjögren's syndrome
- Mixed connective tissue disease

Some clinical features, e.g. Raynaud's phenomenon, arthralgia/arthritis may be present in all, but it is the production of non-organ specific antinuclear antibodies (ANAs) that characterises these diseases. Antibodies to specific nuclear antigens, e.g. anti-double stranded DNA, anti-RO or anti-LA are seen in each disease (see below). Patients occasionally exhibit clinical and serological features of more than one disease, e.g. scleroderma/polymyositis overlap. The vasculitides are often grouped with the connective tissue diseases. This is primarily because the target organ (blood vessels) is a connective tissue. Vasculitis may be a feature of the ANA-associated CTDs. Some of the vasculitides are associated with the production of antineutrophil cytoplasmic antibodies (ANCAs), but many patients with vasculitis produce no autoantibodies.

Autoantibodies: A Synopsis

Antinuclear Antibody

- A simple screening test for connective tissue disease found in:
  - SLE (5% ANA negative), scleroderma, polymyositis, Sjögren's syndrome, mixed connective tissue disease
  - rheumatoid arthritis (RA)
  - autoimmune hepatitis (chronic active hepatitis or primary biliary cirrhosis)
  - also seen with chronic infection and in low titres in normal population
  - titre – the higher the more significant, e.g. > 1 : 160 +

- If ANA positive in a titre of ≥1 : 160, look for antibodies to DS DNA and extractable nuclear antigens (ENA). Among the ENAs are anti-RO, anti-LA, RNP and anti-Sm antibodies

Anti-double-stranded-DNA antibody (DSDNA)

- Elevated in SLE – 70% of patients
- Also RA, chronic active hepatitis, chronic infections, all in low titre
- Titre can act as a guide to disease activity in SLE

Antibodies to Other Nuclear Antigens

- Anti-Ro
  — 75% primary Sjögren's
  — 30% SLE
- Anti-La – less common
  — 50% Sjögren's
  — 10% SLE
- Anti-Sm (Smith) – SLE
- Anti-RNP – mixed connective tissue disease
- Anti-Jo-1 – polymyositis
- Anti-Scl-70 – diffuse scleroderma
- Anti-centromere antibody – limited scleroderma

Antineutrophil Cytoplasmic Antibody

- C-ANCA (cytoplasmic) in Wegener's (high specificity)
- P-ANCA (perinuclear) in microscopic polyarteritis but also present in many inflammatory diseases e.g. inflammatory bowel disease
- The protein recognised by C-ANCA is proteinase 3, by P-ANCA myeloperoxidase.

Anti-phospholipid Antibodies

- see Anti-phospholipid Syndrome (page 75)

Rheumatoid Factor

- Positive in approximately 70% with RA
- Also seen in many chronic diseases, other anti-immune diseases, neoplasia. Present in approximately 4% of normal population

Cryoglobulins

- Immunoglobulins which precipitate and form a gel in the cold. Soluble at body temperature (37°C)
- Must be transported to laboratory at 37°C

- Associated with lymphoproliferative disorders, hepatitis B, C, CMV, SLE, RA
- Clinical features include Raynaud's, arthralgias, vasculitis
- Treat underlying condition, plasmapheresis if severe

Cold Agglutinins

- Immunoglobulins which form a complex with RBCs in cold

Raynaud's Phenomenon

- Reversible vasospasm of peripheral arteries
- Typical colour change white → blue → red (triphasic colour change)
- When severe (usually secondary Raynaud's) can cause ulceration or gangrene of digits

Causes

- Idiopathic
  - F > M
  - age 15–30, prevalence 5–10% of women
- Secondary
  - connective tissue disease
  - RA (10%)
  - drugs – beta-blockers, oral contraceptive pill
  - cryoglobulins
  - vibrating machinery

Indicators of Secondary Raynaud's

- Severe Raynaud's
- Unilateral/asymmetrical
- Rapidly progressive
- Features of underlying disease
- Positive ANA
- Abnormal nailfold capillaroscopy. Dilated, tortuous or absent nailfold capillaries are seen, especially in early scleroderma. Need microscope to view

Exclude Mimics

- Cervical rib, atrial myxoma
- Thromboembolic disease

Management

- Stop smoking
- Calcium channel blockers
- Heated mittens
- Keep core temperature up
- Treat underlying disorder
- IV vasodilators when severe, e.g. prostacyclin infusion
- Cervical or digital sympathectomy
- Consider
  - selective serotonin reuptake inhibitor
  - topical nitroglycerin (applied to any part of skin but not the fingers)
  - opioid analgesics for severe pain (which worsens vasospasm)

Systemic Lupus Erythematosus

- Systemic autoimmune disease with a wide variety of clinical features. Considerable variation in disease severity and organ involvement from mild (most) to life threatening (rare)
- Nine times more common in women than in men

American College of Rheumatology Classification Criteria

Patients must have at least four of the following criteria **in the course** of their disease:

Skin or Mucous Membrane

1 malar rash
2 photosensitivity
3 discoid rash
4 oral ulcers

Locomotor

5 arthritis

Organ Systems

6 serositis – pleuritis or pericarditis
7 renal disorder
8 neurological/psychiatric disorder

Haematological/Serological

9 haematological disorder – haemolytic anaemia/ leucopenia/ lymphopenia/ thrombocytopenia
10 ANA
11 immunological disorder – anti-DSDNA, anti-Sm, anti-phospholipid antibodies

Note

- Many features seen in SLE are not included in the classification criteria, e.g. fatigue, Raynaud's phenomenon, tenosynovitis, fever, signs of vasculitis (rash, livedo reticularis, mononeuritis multiplex), myositis
- Classification criteria are useful for distinguishing one disease from other diseases and for selecting patients for inclusion in clinical studies. They are not diagnostic criteria, as their specificity and sensitivity are less than 100%.

Investigations

- FBC (see 9 above). ↑ ESR
- CRP – normal in SLE flare, raised in infection
- ANA – positive in 95%.
- Anti DSDNA – positive in 50–70%, high specificity for SLE when elevated (titres correlate to a degree with disease activity)
- Complement C_3 and C_4 levels may fall in active disease, especially renal disease
- Coombs test positive
- APTT (if prolonged, check for anti-phospholipid antibodies)
- Urinalysis for protein, urine microscopy for casts and RBCs, urea and electrolytes, creatinine, CPK for myositis
- Chest radiograph, PFTs.
- Measure BP at each visit – onset of renal disease may be insidious
- Not all of the above tests required at each visit – enquire

Management

- Avoid exposure to sunlight, use high-factor sunscreens
- Good education/reassurance
- Drugs
  - NSAIDs for symptomatic relief
  - antimalarial drugs (chloroquine or hydroxychloroquine) for rashes, arthritis and malaise
  - corticosteroids
    - low doses for organ involvement
    - high doses (IV/IM/PO) for severe disease
  - immunosuppressive drugs (azathioprine/ methotrexate/ cyclophosphamide) are generally reserved for involvement of major organs such as kidney, lung, nervous system, vasculitis
- Oestrogen-containing oral contraceptive pill can cause flare of SLE. Use progesterone-only pill if necessary

If the Patient is Pregnant

- Check anticardiolipin antibodies and lupus anticoagulant. Low-dose aspirin if antibody positive or history of first trimester fetal loss. Subcutaneous heparin if there is a history of late fetal loss
- Pre-eclampsia is a frequent complication of pregnancy in lupus. There is an increased incidence of fetal death in late pregnancy. One in four pregnancies ends in fetal loss
- Check anti-RO as antibodies can cross placenta and cause heart block in foetus
- Inform obstetrician

Additional Treatments

- for hypertension
- for infection
- for cerebral lupus (anticonvulsant)
- for thrombosis (heparin/ warfarin)
- for haematological disorders (splenectomy occasionally)

Drug-induced Lupus

S   sulfonamides (including sulfasalazine)
H   hydralazine
O   oral contraceptive pill (contraindicated in systemic lupus)
P   phenothiazines/procainamide
A   anticonvulsants:
    — phenytoin
    — carbamazepine
T   tetracyclines

Features

- ANA positive
- DSDNA negative
- Renal/CNS involvement unusual
- Resolves on drug withdrawal

Anti-phospholipid Syndrome (APS)

Clinical Features (mnemonic "CLOT")

C venous/arterial thrombosis (clotting) e.g. DVT, stroke, transient ischaemic attack
L livedo reticularis (lace-like rash on extremities)
O obstetric loss, usually mid trimester
T thrombocytopenia
- Leg ulcers, cardiac valve lesions also occur
- APS is diagnosed if there is a history of thrombosis, obstetric loss or thrombocytopenia in the presence of anticardiolipin antibodies or lupus anticoagulant
- Cardiolipin antibodies: IgM or IgG must be present on two occasions 3 months apart
- Lupus anticoagulant is present when APTT is prolonged (in absence of heparin treatment), and when APTT is not correctable by addition of normal plasma. Coagulation problem is therefore due to the presence of an inhibitor of coagulation.
- If anticardiolipin negative but APS strongly suspected, check for anti-beta 2 glycoprotein 1 antibodies. Beta 2 glycoprotein 1 is an anticoagulant protein. Those who are anticardiolipin positive due to infection but who are beta 2 glycoprotein 1 antibody negative are not at increased risk of thrombosis.
- APS may be:
  — primary – no other disease
  — secondary – e.g. SLE, infections, hepatitis

Treatment

- Low dose aspirin usually if antibody positive only
- Lifelong warfarin for arterial or venous thrombosis (keep INR 3.0–4.0)
- Oral steroids for severe thrombocytopenia

Mixed Connective Tissue Disease (MCTD)

- Features of a number of CTDs in one patient
- Associated antibodies to ribonucleoprotein (RNP)
- Antibodies to DSDNA, SCL 70, etc. absent
- Renal/CNS disease rare; lung (pulmonary fibrosis/pulmonary hypertension) more common
- Treat clinical features as appropriate

Some rheumatologists prefer the term "undifferentiated connective tissue disease" and do not recognise MCTD as a specific entity.

Sjögren's Syndrome

- Inflammatory autoimmune disease affecting primarily exocrine glands
- Female to male ratio 9 : 1
- Onset 40–60 years

Classification

- Primary Sjögren's – absence of another autoimmune disease (30%)
- Secondary Sjögren's – evidence of other autoimmune disease, e.g. RA, connective tissue disease, or organ specific autoimmune diseases e.g. pernicious anaemia, thyroid disease, liver disease

Features

- Xerophthalmia (dry eyes)
- Xerostomia (dry mouth)
- Dyspareunia
- Arthralgia/arthritis
- Parotid gland enlargement
- Raynaud's phenomenon
- ↑ incidence of lymphoma (check for lymphadenopathy, hepatosplenomegaly)
- Hypothyroidism
- Uncommon – pulmonary fibrosis, peripheral neuropathy, renal tubular acidosis

Investigation

- ESR usually raised
- FBC anaemia, leucopenia, thrombocytopenia
- ↑ globulin fraction (check every 1–2 years, falling globulins or monoclonal band on electrophoresis are clues to developing lymphoma)
- Autoantibodies:
  — rheumatoid factor positive in 80–90%
  — ANF positive in 90%
  — anti-Ro positive in 70–90%
  — anti-La positive in 40–50%
- Thyroid function tests
- Chest radiograph – pulmonary fibrosis (uncommon)
- Schirmer's test:
  — filter paper 30 mm in length, slipped beneath lower eyelid
  — test is positive if less than 5 mm of paper is wet after 5 minutes

- Salivary gland biopsy:
  - biopsy minor lip glands
  - evidence of lymphocytic infiltration on histology
- Rose Bengal staining of conjunctiva

Treatment: (mainly symptomatic)

- Dry eyes
  - artificial tears
- Dry mouth
  - sugar-free lozenges
  - good dental care
  - treatment of oral candida
  - pilocarpine tablets
- Arthritis
  - NSAIDs
  - hydroxychloroquine
  - low dose steroids
- Severe disease, e.g. renal impairment, may require high dose corticosteroids or immunosuppressive drugs such as cyclophosphamide or azathioprine
- In general avoid immunosuppression due to existing ↑ risk of lymphoma

Scleroderma

- Rare connective tissue disorder. Female to male ratio 4 : 1, onset age 30–50
- Two main clinical presentations:
  - **limited scleroderma**: upper arms and legs and trunk spared = CREST syndrome (calcinosis, Raynaud's, esophageal dysmotility, sclerodactyly, telangiectasia)
  - **diffuse scleroderma**: widespread skin thickening, high frequency of internal organ involvement especially lung, heart, GIT, renal = systemic sclerosis
- Positive ANA in both:
  - anti-centromere antibodies (limited)
  - anti-Scl70 (diffuse)

Assessment

- Measure BP monthly (increasing BP predicts onset of scleroderma renal crisis in diffuse scleroderma)
- Chest radiograph, PFTs, high-resolution CT thorax (in diffuse) to look for alveolitis fibrosis
- ECG, ECHO annually. Pulmonary hypertension occurs in both limited and diffuse
- CPK (myositis)
- Weight, serum albumin (malabsorbtion)
- U&E, creatinine

Management

- Keep body core temperature up (not just hands warm)
- Treat skin infections promptly
- Calcium channel blocker for Raynaud's
- Prostacyclin IV for severe Raynaud's (pain or digital ischaemia)
- Proton pump inhibitor for heartburn
- ACE inhibitor if BP ↑ (protects against renal crisis)
- Rotating antibiotics for malabsorption secondary to bacterial overgrowth
- Consider IV cyclophosphamide for alveolitis
- Avoid high-dose steroids (>20 mg prednisolone daily) – risk of precipitating scleroderma renal crisis
- Losartan for pulmonary hypertension

Polymyositis/Dermatomyositis

- Uncommon inflammatory disease of muscle. In dermatomyositis (DM)– heliotrope (purple rash) on eyelids and rash around PIPs, MCPs

(Gottron's papules). Rash may precede muscle weakness by months. Some develop a macular rash around neck/shoulder girdle "shawl sign". Calcinosis can occur in juvenile DM
- Insidious onset of muscle weakness. Diffuse, symmetrical, predominantly proximal

Investigations

- ↑↑ CPK/aldolase
- Myositis on muscle biopsy
- Whole body MRI may be very useful to document site for biopsy, extent of disease and response to treatment
- Characteristic EMG abnormality
- 80% ANA positive. Anti-Jo1 antibodies positive in 25%.
- Anti-synthetase antibodies (Jo1) positivity is associated with ↑ risk of interstitial lung disease
- Dermatomyositis is associated with underlying malignancy in about 20% of cases. Limited screening for malignancy worthwhile in dermatomyositis, e.g. chest radiograph, abdominal and pelvic ultrasound, tumour markers, urinalysis, faecal occult bloods, prostate-specific antigen

Treatment

- Needs to be treated early and aggressively
- Steroids (1 mg/kg daily initially)
- Steroid-sparing agents – methotrexate/azathioprine/cyclosporine
- Muscle strengthening exercises

Differential Diagnosis of Muscle Pain and or Weakness

Infectious Diseases

- Viral, e.g. influenza, hepatitis B and C, HIV
- Bacterial, e.g. Lyme disease, pyomyositis
- Other, e.g. toxoplasmosis, cysticercosis

Auto-immune Diseases

- PM/DM, SLE, Sjögren's, scleroderma
- Vasculitis
- Polymyalgia rheumatica
- Myasthenia gravis

Drug Induced

- Alcohol
- Lipid lowering agents
- Hydroxychloroquine
- Colchicine
- Cimetidine
- With rhabdomyolosis (acute, CPK ↑↑↑, myoglobinuria) – alcohol, cocaine, heroin, neuroleptics, anaesthetics (e.g. halothane)

Endocrine/Metabolic Diseases

- Cushing's syndrome, hyper- and hypothyroidism, hypocalcaemia, hypokalaemia

Others

- Carcinoma
- Inclusion body myositis
- Fibromyalgia
- Neurological diseases
- Muscular dystrophies
- Congenital myopathies

The above list is not exhaustive but offers a template for investigation of muscle disorders, in particular objective muscle weakness. Discuss the extent and sequence of investigations with the rheumatologist. Neurological opinion is often helpful.

Vasculitis

- Inflammatory disease involving blood vessels
- Uncommon or rare
- The most common clinical presentation is cutaneous vasculitis. The aim of investigation is to:
  - look for evidence of involvement of other systems
  - find the cause
  - exclude mimics of vasculitis, e.g. atrial myxoma, subacute bacterial endocarditis

Classification

Classified according to size of vessel involved:

- Small vessel
  - Henoch–Schonlein purpura
  - hypersensitivity vasculitis

- drugs
  - infections e.g. hepatitis B or C, HIV
- microscopic polyarteritis
- connective tissue disease
  - RA
  - lupus
  - Sjögren's syndrome
  - cryoglobulinaemia
- malignancy
- medium vessel
  - polyarteritis nodosa (PAN)
  - Wegener's granulomatosis
  - Churg–Strauss syndrome
- Large vessel
  - giant cell (temporal) arteritis
  - Takayasu's arteritis

Henoch–Schonlein Purpura

- Characterised by IgA deposition in small vessels
- Cutaneous vasculitis, abdominal pain, arthritis and renal disease are the principal clinical features
- Acute, usually self limiting
- More common in children

Microscopic Polyarteritis (MPA)

- Focal segmental necrotising small vessel vasculitis
- Glomerulonephritis common
- Does not cause microaneurysm formation
- P-ANCA usually positive but no granuloma formation

Polyarteritis Nodosa (PAN)

- Focal segmental necrotising medium vessel vasculitis
- Usually involves skin, kidney, muscle, nerve and GI tract
- Microaneurysms on magnetic resonance angiogram
- Some cases are associated with hepatitis B

Wegener's Granulomatosis (WG)

- Rare, granulomatous medium vessel vasculitis
- Involves upper airways, lower respiratory tract, kidney, eye and skin
- C-ANCA positivity is ~90% specific for WG

Churg–Strauss Syndrome (CSS)

- Rare granulomatous small and medium vessel vasculitis
- Strongly associated with a history of allergy e.g. rhinitis, asthma
- Pronounced peripheral and tissue eosinophilia
- P-ANCA positive

Note

Five-year survival for MPA, PAN, WG and CSS is approximately 70%.

Takayasu's Arteritis

- Large vessel panarteritis
- Most commonly occurs in young females
- Aortic arch and abdominal aorta most commonly affected
- Diagnose on MR or contrast angiography

Investigations

- FBC, ESR
- RF, ANA, ANCA
- U&E, creatinine, CPK
- Cryoglobulins, serum protein electrophoresis, C_3C_4
- Hepatitis screen (25% of PAN patients hepatitis B positive, hepatitis C positive in cryoglobulinaemia)
- Skin/muscle/organ biopsy/sural or superficial peroneal nerve biopsy
- Urinalysis (spun for granular or red cell casts)
- Chest radiograph
- Echocardiogram, cholesterol, anti-glomerular basement membrane antibodies
- Nerve conduction studies
- Angiogram (contrast or MR)

Treatment

- Depends on severity and extent of organ involvement. See local protocols
- Corticosteroids, methotrexate, cyclophosphamide, azathioprine, IV immune globulin, mycophenylate mofetil. Colchicine occasionally for cutaneous vasculitis

Infection and Arthritis   **14**

A number of bacteria and viruses can cause arthritis. Fungal arthritis usually occurs only in immunocompromised patients. Lyme disease (see below) is caused by a spirochaete.

Bacterial Septic Arthritis (Non-gonococcal)

- Is a medical emergency. Most commonly due to *Staphylococcus aureus* (up to 50% of cases); *Staphylococcus epidermidis*, streptococci, gram-negative bacteria and anaerobes account for the remainder of cases
- Bacteria reach a joint via haematogenous spread, direct penetration through skin or by local spread from an adjacent infected site
- Clinical features include signs of acute monoarthritis with marked constitutional symptoms, e.g. fever, rigors. Classic signs may be absent in elderly or immunocompromised patients. A high index of clinical suspicion is necessary
- Prosthetic joints, joints damaged by chronic arthritis (e.g. rheumatoid arthritis, haemarthrosis, osteoarthritis) are at increased risk of infection. Impaired host defence due to neoplastic disease or chronic severe illness (diabetes, cirrhosis, chronic renal disease, HIV) and immune suppression with steroids or chemotherapy are well-known risk factors
- Management includes prompt diagnosis by repeated blood cultures, skin swabs if relevant, aspiration of joint and Gram's stain and culture of synovial fluid
- Broad-spectrum antibiotics should be commenced while awaiting culture and sensitivity results. A combination of IV penicillin with a third-generation cephalosporin is recommended. If enterococci are suspected, cephalosporins may be replaced with gentamicin. Give parenteral antibiotics for 1–2 weeks and for a total of 4–6 weeks. Rest affected joint until inflammation subsides. Surgical drainage of the joint may be necessary
- Falling serum CRP and WCC in synovial fluid useful for monitoring early response

- Infected prosthetic joints in most cases must be removed
- Intra-articular steroids are contraindicated where sepsis is suspected

Gonococcal Arthritis

- Infection with *Neisseria gonorrhoeae* is sexually transmitted
- Arthritis occurs in 1–3%
- Common clinical features include tenosynovitis, dermatitis (maculopapular/vesicular/pustular rash), and migratory polyarthralgia with or without purulent arthritis
- Diagnosis: sexual history (for venereal disease risk), clinical examination (pustules/tenosynovitis), and laboratory analysis of blood cultures, synovial fluid Gram's stain and culture, skin and/or urethral swabs
- Treatment is recommended with ceftriaxone or cefotaxime. In penicillin-allergic patients, quinolones can be used. Duration of therapy 7–14 days. Patients also require joint drainage with repeated aspiration
- Patients should be screened for syphilis and HIV. Sexual partners should be screened for gonorrhoea and other venereal diseases

Tuberculosis

- Usually mono-articular or mono-osseous. Common sites are spine, hip, knee, ankle or sacroiliac joint. Osteomyelitis can affect any long bone
- Onset insidious and slowly progressive. Constitutional symptoms, e.g. fatigue, weight loss, fever with night sweats common
- Risk factors include alcoholism, pre-existing joint disease and prolonged use of steroids and/or immune suppression
- Diagnosis: acid-fast bacilli or TB culture of biopsy material. Standard anti-TB treatment should be used and prolonged surveillance after treatment is needed

Brucellosis and Arthritis

- Zoonotic infection. Well-recognised cause of fever of unknown origin. Onset can be abrupt or insidious
- One-third may develop a focal osteoarticular complication, especially sacroiliitis. Diagnosis is often delayed. Should be considered in unexplained arthritis, particularly sacroiliitis
- Diagnosis is established by culture, serology and/or polymerase chain reaction
- Treatment is usually with doxycycline + streptomycin/gentamicin or doxycycline + rifampicin

Lyme Disease

- Caused by spirochaete *Borrelia burgdorferi*: infection is tick-borne
- The tick vector, *Ixodes*, is found on rodents in wooded, brush or grassy areas
- Children under the age of 15 years and middle-aged adults have highest incidence
- Clinical features are divided into three stages:
  1 early localised disease characterized by erythema migrans (a red macule/papule more than 5 cm with central clearing) and constitutional symptoms
  2 early disseminated disease: neurologic and/or cardiac manifestations usually after weeks or months after infection.
  3 late Lyme disease with intermittent acute/chronic arthritis and/or neurological problems developing weeks to years later
- Isolation of spirochaete from tissue or body fluid or detection of diagnostic levels of antibodies establishes diagnosis in serum or CSF. False positive results may occur with ELISA testing in other infections such as syphilis. Western blot test for confirmation
- Treat early localised disease with amoxycillin or doxycycline or cefuroxime for 3 weeks. Arthritis, a manifestation of early, disseminated disease or late Lyme disease is best treated with ceftriaxone or cefotaxime. A minority of patients may have refractory disease

Viral Arthritis

- A number of viruses can cause arthritis. Generally the arthritis occurs during the viral prodrome, is non-destructive and does not lead to chronic joint disease
- Common viruses associated with arthritis include human parvovirus (HPV) B19, hepatitis B and C, rubella and HIV
- Human parvovirus B19, a single-stranded DNA virus, is transmitted by respiratory secretions and occasionally by contaminated blood products
  — acute symmetrical polyarthritis in hands and wrists
  — can mimic adult or juvenile rheumatoid arthritis. symptoms are self-limiting, but may persist for months
  — diagnosis: B19 IgM antibodies or viral B19 DNA. IgG antibodies of little significance as they persist for years
- HIV infection is associated with a number of rheumatic syndromes and should be considered in-patients with risk factors for HIV infection. They include:
  — articular: arthralgia, reiter's syndrome, psoriatic arthritis, undifferentiated spondylarthropathy, HIV-induced arthritis and painful articular syndrome

- muscular: myalgia, polymyositis, and myopathy
- diffuse infiltrative lymphocytosis syndrome (DILS)
- vasculitis
- infection: septic arthritis, osteomyelitis, pyomyositis

Pregnancy and Rheumatic Diseases   **15**

Before Pregnancy

- If a patient tells you she has become pregnant or is considering pregnancy, ask the rheumatologist to see her
- Female patients on methotrexate, leflunomide or cyclophosphamide should not attempt to become pregnant; a male patient should not attempt to father a child. The drugs are potentially teratogenic
- Women on biologic agents (e.g. etanercept, anakinra, infliximab) should use adequate contraception as the effects on the foetus are unknown
- Sulfasalazine, methotrexate and azathioprine may reduce the sperm count and thus fertility
- Women with active inflammatory arthritis appear less likely to become pregnant that than those whose arthritis is inactive
- Those starting cyclophosphamide should consider sperm or ovum banking

During Pregnancy

Ideally all drugs should be stopped, but this may not be feasible. For many rheumatic diseases the effect of pregnancy cannot be predicted (may be better or worse). In rheumatoid arthritis >50% will improve during pregnancy, with relapse occurring some weeks after delivery.

Drugs

- Paracetamol
  - safe
  - usual doses
- NSAIDs
  - not teratogenic
  - can cause oligohydramnios
  - stop in late pregnancy (risk of early closure of ductus arteriosus)
  - can prolong labour and cause excessive bleeding

- low dose aspirin, e.g. for antiphospholipid syndrome, safe in late pregnancy/delivery
- Corticosteroids
  - safe
  - consider calcium/vitamin D supplements
- Hydroxychloroquine
  - no excess of birth abnormalities
  - used especially in SLE
- Sulfasalazine
  - frequently continued during pregnancy if needed
- Azathioprine
  - no excess of birth abnormalities
- Methotrexate, leflunomide, cyclophosphamide
  - dangerous during pregnancy
  - avoid
  - see above
- Cyclosporin
  - many successful pregnancies in transplant patients
- Myocrisin
  - crosses placenta but appears safe
- Etanercept, infliximab, anakinra
  - limited experience to date, but some successful pregnancies with no birth defects

After Childbirth

- Most patients are advised to restart their previous medication. This may not apply where the mother is breast-feeding
- Methotrexate, leflunomide, cyclophosphamide, cyclosporin and myocrisin must not be taken while breast-feeding
- Sulfasalazine and hydroxychloroquine have been used successfully while breast-feeding
- Corticosteroids are excreted in small amounts in breast milk but are probably safe in small doses
- NSAIDs can be safely used but doses should be kept as low as possible. High dose aspirin is excreted in breast milk and should be avoided

Inheritance and Rheumatic Diseases   **16**

Patients are often worried about the chances of passing their condition on to their children. The following information may be helpful.

Rheumatoid Arthritis

- May cluster within families but more commonly sporadic
- Slightly increased risk in female offspring of an affected mother, less for male offspring
- Risk of RA in identical twin if one twin affected is 1 in 6, for non-identical twin 1 in 20 (same as for siblings)

Osteoarthritis

- Large joint OA (e.g. hip, knee): heredity usually a small risk factor.
- Nodal OA DIP/PIP/1st CMC: if mother has nodal OA, there is a 1 in 2 chance of daughter inheriting it

Ankylosing Spondylitis

- If a patient has ankylosing spondylitis and is B27 positive, the risk of a child being B27 positive is 1 in 2. The risk of a B27 positive relative of a patient with AS developing AS themselves is 1 in 3. Therefore overall risk of a child of AS patient developing AS is approximately 1 in 6

Sytemic Lupus Erythematosus (SLE)

- If a patient has SLE, the risk of a child developing it is approximately 1 in 100. The risk for a sibling of a patient is higher (approximately 1 in 33)
- If a patient is RO antibody positive there is a 1 in 20 risk of the child developing congenital heart block

Crystal Arthritis 17

Two common conditions are associated with crystal deposition in joints:

- gout
- pseudogout

Gout

- Acute inflammatory arthritis that affects peripheral joints with deposition of monosodium urate crystals in and around joints and tendons
- Usually affects 1–2 joints (oligoarticular) but may be polyarticular
- Most commonly affects 1st MTP joint (podagra)
- Also affects mid-tarsal joints, ankle, knee, wrist
- Joints are usually warm, red, tender and swollen with overlying shiny skin
- Repeated attacks may lead to bone erosion
- Factors that may precipitate attack:
  - trauma
  - infection
  - surgery
  - stress
  - alcohol
  - drugs (e.g. thiazide)

Investigation

- Joint aspiration – needle-shaped crystals of monosodium urate which show negative birefringence in polarised light
- Blood tests
  - serum urate – usually raised, but may be normal even in an acute attack
  - FBC – to screen for polycythaemia rubra vera (rare), macrocytosis (alcohol)

— Urea and Electrolytes – urate nephropathy (uncommon)
— fasting lipids – type IV hyperlipidaemia is associated with gout
- Liver function tests
- Radiographs – punched out lesions with overhanging edges, soft tissue swelling. Urate stones in urinary tract are not radio-opaque

Treatment

- NSAIDs in full dose
- Intra-articular steroid for confirmed gouty monoarthropathy
- Oral steroid course if not responsive to NSAIDs. Dosage – crash course "asthma style" for 10 days, initially 30–40 mg per day falling to zero

Allopurinol

- Indications:
  — tophaceous gout
  — recurrent attacks > 4 per year
- Dosage:
  — initially 100–200 mg once daily increasing weekly to maintenance 200–400 mg
  — commence allopurinol 10–14 days after acute attack subsides
  — aim to keep serum urate in **lower half** of the normal range
  — reduce dose in elderly patient or renal impairment (100–200 mg/day maximum)
- Asymptomatic hyperuricaemia is not an indication for allopurinol.
- **Remember**: dangerous interaction between allopurinol and azathioprine – avoid co-prescription
- Colchicine rarely used for acute attacks due to GI side effects. Low dose 0.5 mg twice daily may be useful for prophylaxis
- Dietician referral (reduce protein intake, weight reduction, low fat as appropriate)
- Advice regarding reducing alcohol intake
- Do not stop allopurinol if a breakthrough attack occurs. Use full dose NSAID, oral steroids or low dose oral colchicine and maintain allopurinol

Pseudogout

"Little old lady disease"

- Calcium pyrophosphate crystal deposition disease (CPPD)
- Crystals deposited in cartilage
- Shedding of crystals into joint space provokes an acute attack of synovitis known as pseudogout
- Patients may experience acute or subacute attacks of arthritis that affect typically the knee, wrist or MCP joint
- Associated with hypothyroidism, gout, haemochromatosis, hypomagnasaemia
- Often have underlying osteoarthritis

Investigations

- Joint aspiration –calcium pyrophosphate crystals with positive birefringence in polarised light
- Radiographs– chondrocalcinosis, especially knee, triangular cartilage at wrist
- Ferritin – to exclude haemochromatosis
- Bone profile – to exclude hyperparathyroidism
- Urate – to exclude gout
- Thyroid function tests
- Magnesium

Treatment

- NSAIDs
- Intra-articular steroid injection
- Short course of oral steroid if acute attack fails to respond to NSAIDs (similar to gout)

Polymyalgia Rheumatica (PMR) **18**

- Inflammatory condition occurring typically in patients > 60 years
- More common in women, occasionally associated with giant cell arteritis (GCA) = temporal arteritis
- Usually associated with ↑↑ ESR (at least > 40 mm/h)
- Onset can be dramatic or insidious

History

- Marked proximal pain and stiffness (bilateral, hip and shoulder girdles, difficulty combing hair, getting out of a chair)
- Fatigue, malaise, anorexia
- Depression
- Weight loss
- Headaches, scalp tenderness, visual disturbance, jaw claudication. The presence of any of these symptoms raises the possibility of GCA

Examination

- Muscle strength normal (but may be reduced by pain)
- Pain on joint movement
- Restriction of shoulder movement if diagnosis is delayed
- Small joint involvement can occur infrequently, e.g. wrist, MCP. Knee, ankle or MTP involvement is more suggestive of late onset rheumatoid arthritis
- Temporal artery tenderness/soft tissue swelling/absent pulse in GCA

Investigation

- Bloods:
  — ESR ↑↑
  — FBC – normochromic anaemia
  — alkaline phosphatase may be elevated

— RF – if positive in high titre, raises the likelihood of rheumatoid arthritis
— CPK to exclude myositis (but myositis usually not painful)

Management

- Oral steroids (PMR 15–20 mg/day, taper slowly, GCA 60 mg/day, taper slowly) Treat suspected GCA urgently. Permanent visual loss can occur if untreated
- Response is characteristically rapid (days). Reduce dose while monitoring symptoms and ESR
- Many require steroid therapy for 2 years or longer. Use osteoporosis prophylaxis

Osteoporosis 19

- Reduction in total or regional bone mass resulting in predisposition to skeletal fractures. Reduction in mass is greater than expected for normal ageing process
- Increased risk of wrist, vertebral and hip fracture in particular
- Common, underdiagnosed and undertreated

Risk Factors

- Family history
- Low calcium intake
- Low body mass
- Sedentary lifestyle
- Corticosteroids (maximum bone mass loss is in first weeks of treatment)
- Cigarette smoking
- Early menopause
- Excessive alcohol consumption
- Previous low trauma fracture
- History of falls

Investigations

- Radiography is unreliable for the assessment of bone density. Osteopenia on radiographs correlates poorly with bone mineral density as measured by DEXA
- Bone chemistry normal
- Check serum testosterone in men

DEXA Scan (dual energy X-ray absorptiometry)

The **T score** is the number of standard deviations that a patient's value is above or below the mean peak value for young adults:

- between −1 and −2.5 = osteopenia
- below −2.5 = osteoporosis

Lumbar spine T score may be underestimated by degenerative changes. The T score threshold for intervention in steroid-induced osteoporosis should be lower than for postmenopausal osteoporosis.

- T score of –1 increases fracture risk × 2
- T score of –2 increases fracture risk × 4
- T score of –3 increases fracture risk × 8, etc.
- Previous low trauma fracture further doubles risk

The **Z score** is the number of standard deviations that a patient's value is above or below the mean value for age matched adults (ZAMA).

Indications for DEXA Scan

- Maintenance steroids (3 months or longer)
- Risk factors, as above (2 or more factors present)
- Monitoring response to therapy

Management

- Ensure adequate calcium and vitamin D intake
- Encourage weight bearing and resistance exercise
- Reduce alcohol intake, stop smoking
- Fracture prevention advice
- Reduce or eliminate any factors associated with falling, e.g. postural hypotension, poor balance, impaired vision in elderly
- Bisphosphonates
  - etidronate (weak) – less commonly used now; evidence for reduction in vertebral fractures only
  - risedronate (potent) – fast acting, reduces vertebral and hip fractures
  - alendronate (potent) – once weekly preparation convenient; reduces vertebral and hip fractures
  - note: biosphosphonates are poorly absorbed from the gastro-intestinal tract. Patients need to fast for at least 30 minutes before and after taking the drug. It should be taken with a generous amount of water (100 ml) and patients should not lie down for at least 30 minutes after taking it. These measures reduce upper GI intolerance, including oesophageal ulceration
  - women of child-bearing age must use contraceptive measures if taking a bisphosphonate
  - correct duration of therapy is unknown but minimum likely to be 3–5 years
- Hormone replacement therapy: Evidence of reduction in vertebral fractures. Increased risk of breast cancer with long-term use and consequent restricted duration of therapy reduces its effectiveness in osteoporosis

- SERM (selective oestrogen receptor modulator), e.g. raloxifene:
  — reduces incidence of vertebral fractures but no hip data
  — no increase in risk of breast cancer (the opposite is more likely) but cannot be used for menopausal symptoms, e.g. flushes, sweats
  — main indication is in age group 55–70 at risk of vertebral fracture
  — not licensed for steroid-induced osteoporosis.
- Hip protectors in elderly patients, e.g. nursing home residents
- Steroid-induced osteoporosis
  — all patients on oral steroids should take calcium and vitamin D supplements
  — if likely to be on oral steroids e.g. prednisolone 5 mg daily or greater for 3 months, add bisphosphonate (alendronate or risedronate)

Acute Vertebral Fracture

- Most acute vertebral fractures are relatively asymptomatic and do not come to medical attention
- Some acute fractures present with severe thoracic or lumbar pain and reduced mobility. The typical patient is thin, elderly and female with pre-existing vertebral fractures
- Potent analgesics may be required initially, e.g. tramadol, oxycodone, fentanyl patch
- Salmon calcitonin 10 mg SC (test dose) followed by 80–100 u daily may ease bone pain but nausea is frequent
- Maximise osteoporosis treatment
- Physiotherapy to restore mobility

Paget's Disease

- Common condition (5% of older population) but frequently asymptomatic
- Abnormal bone turnover results in remodelling of bone shape and size
- Bony pelvis, femur and skull most frequently affected
- Radiographs demonstrate altered bone architecture, bone sclerosis and disorganised trabecular structure
- Although many cases asymptomatic, may cause bone pain. Increased risk of fracture and nerve, cord or brain compression. Osteosarcoma (0.1%) is a rare complication

Investigation

- Plain radiograph
- Alkaline phosphatase ↑ (correlates with activity)
- Calcium, phosphate normal
- Urinary hydroxyproline ↑

Management

- No intervention in absence of pain or risk of neurological compromise
- Pain, potential bone deformity (e.g. femur, tibia) or neurological abnormality are indications for treatment
- Reducing bone turnover before replacing a pagetic hip is a further possible indication

Drug Treatment

- A range of bisphosphonates are used, including:
  — etidronate 5 mg/kg daily × 6 months
  — alendronate 40 mg daily × 3 months
  — risedronate 30 mg daily × 2 months
  — pamidronate 60 mg IV every 3 months as indicated

- Resolution of symptoms, normalisation of alkaline phosphatase indicate a response to treatment. Further courses of treatment may be given for relapses

Osteomalacia 21

- Defective mineralisation of bone resulting in a reduction in ratio of mineralised bone to bone matrix
- Most common causes are vitamin D deficiency or acquired defects in vitamin D metabolism

Common Causes

- Causes of vitamin D deficiency
  - poor diet (especially elderly, alcohol abuse)
  - inadequate sun exposure
  - malabsorption
- Acquired causes of abnormal vitamin D metabolism
  - chronic liver disease
  - chronic renal disease
  - anticonvulsant drugs

Less Common/Rare Causes

- Congenital causes of abnormal vitamin D metabolism
  - X-linked hypophosphataemic rickets
  - vitamin D dependent rickets
  - renal tubular acidosis
- Oncogenic osteomalacia
  - severe hypophosphataemia associated with osteomalacia secondary to malignancy

Symptoms

- Bone pain
- Proximal muscle weakness
- Bone deformities (in children)

Investigations

- Serum calcium low
- Serum phosphate low
- Alkaline phosphatase raised
- 25 OH-vitamin D low

Plain radiographs – pseudofractures or Looser's zones – incomplete fracture lines at right angles to the cortex, especially at pubic rami, femoral neck, ribs

Treatment

- Vitamin D and calcium supplements for dietary deficiency or malabsorption. Dose depends on the cause. Chronic renal failure – seek specialist advice

Uncommon Rheumatological Conditions 22

Reflex Sympathetic Dystrophy (RSD)

- Also known as algodystrophy
- Poorly understood condition
- Clinical features include pain (often severe), diffuse and marked tenderness, soft tissue swelling. Warmth over affected part and localised sweating are also seen. Hand and foot most commonly affected. Occasionally can affect hip or knee
- Triggered by trauma (accident, burn, surgery, etc.), hemiplegia, meningitis, pregnancy, tumours, prolonged immobilization. In a quarter of patients no clear trigger identified. In some, psychological factors have a role
- The diagnosis is essentially clinical. Triple-phase technetium scintigraphy may be helpful, also MRI
- Management includes reassurance and counselling, antidepressants, pain management including transcutaneous nerve stimulation, regional sympathetic or ganglion block. Encourage use of affected limb

Relapsing Polychondritis

- Disease of unknown cause characterised by episodic and sometimes progressive cartilage inflammation
- Ear, nose, larynx, joints, heart and eyes are common sites of involvement
- Underlying systemic rheumatic illness e.g. (RA, SLE, Sjögren's syndrome) seen in some patients
- Diagnosis is clinical
- Management options include NSAIDs, dapsone, and steroids in systemic disease

Pigmented Villonodular Synovitis (PVNS)

- Rare non-malignant condition characterised by dramatic synovial hypertrophy
- Cause unknown. Presents as a monoarthritis or monotenosynovitis. Knee most common site. Usual age 20–40 years
- Gradual onset pain and swelling in the absence of trauma is the usual presentation
- Diagnosis is by synovial biopsy. MRI may suggest the diagnosis
- Is associated with bleeding in the joint space: synovial aspirate often sero-sanguinous
- Management: surgical or radiation synovectomy and occasionally arthroplasty

Rheumatic Fever

- Immunological sequel to group A streptococcal pharyngeal infection. Manifests after a latent period of 2–3 weeks after infection
- Diagnosis is based on revised Jones criteria: A firm diagnosis requires two major manifestations or one major and two minor manifestations along with evidence of recent streptococcal infection
- Major manifestations: carditis, polyarthritis, chorea, erythema marginatum and subcutaneous nodules
- Minor manifestations: fever, arthralgia, previous rheumatic fever or rheumatic heart disease
- Tests:
  - FBC: usually shows normocytic normochromic anaemia
  - ESR is increased
  - Anti-streptolysin O titre is increased; falls rapidly (in weeks)
  - Throat swab for group A beta-haemolytic streptococci
  - ECG: increased P–R interval
- Management includes anti-inflammatory agent, usually aspirin, a course of penicillin for 10 days, even in absence of pharyngitis, steroids for carditis. Long-term penicillin prophylaxis with oral penicillin V 250 000 i.u. twice a day or Penicillin G 1.2 million i.u. intramuscularly every 3–4 weeks should be given for patients who have had rheumatic fever. Erythromycin 250 mg daily may be used in patients allergic to penicillin

Adult Onset Still's Disease (AOSD)

- Characterised by daily high fever (>39°C), arthritis and evanescent rash
- Clinical and laboratory features similar to systemic onset juvenile chronic arthritis
- Majority of cases manifest between age 16–34 years
- Laboratory features include elevated ESR, increased WCC (>15000 × 10^9/L) normocytic normochromic anaemia, and elevated transaminases. Markedly elevated serum ferritin (greater than 5 × normal limit) is seen in about 70% of patients
- The disease course can be self-limiting, intermittent or chronic
- Treatment includes NSAIDs or aspirin. Steroids for debilitating joint symptoms, high fever or internal organ involvement. Traditional DMARDs may be needed

Sarcoidosis

- Multisystem disease, aetiology unknown, characterised histologically by non-caseating granuloma formation
- Musculoskeletal manifestations
  - acute periarthritis associated with erythema nodosum and bihilar adenopathy
  - usually involves ankle or knee
  - swelling, erythema around affected joint
  - resolves in weeks
  - can also cause chronic arthropathy, bone cysts and dactylitis (uncommon, 5%)
  - granulomatous muscle involvement can occur in acute sarcoid
- Intra-articular or oral steroid may be required in acute cases

Further Reading

Klippel J, Dieppe P, eds, *Rheumatology*, 2nd edition. London: Mosby, 1998

West SG, *Rheumatology Secrets*, 2nd edition. Philadelphia: Hanley and Belfus, 2002

Doherty M, Hazleman BL, Hutson CW, Maddison PJ, Perry JD, *Rheumatology Examination and Injection Techniques*, 2nd edition. London: Harcourt Brace, 1999

Useful Websites

Medscape Rheumatology
www.medscape.com/rheumatologyhome

Rheumatologyweb
www.rheumatologyweb.com

International League of Associations for Rheumatology (ILAR)
www.ilar.org

American College of Rheumatology (ACR)
www.rheumatology.org

Arthritis Rheumatism Campaign (ARC)
www.arc.org.uk

Irish Society for Rheumatology (ISR)
www.isr.i.e.

British Society for Rheumatology
www.rheumatology.org.uk

European League Against Rheumatism (EULAR)
www.eular.org

Index

A
Achilles bursitis, 15
Achilles tear, 15
Achilles tendonitis, 15, 52
Acromioclavicular joint pain, 14
Adhesive capsulitis, 14, 47
Admission to hospital, 23
Allopurinol, 91
American College of Rheumatology
    Classification criteria
        rheumatoid arthritis, 60
        systemic lupus erythematosus, 72
    indices, 22
Anakinra, 37
Analgesics, 27–8
Ankle pain, 15
Ankylosing spondylitis, 10, 14, 64–6
    inheritance, 89
Anterior chest wall pain, 14
Anti-double-stranded-DNA antibody, 70
Anti-phospholipid syndrome, 75
Antineutrophil cytoplasmic antibody, 70
Antinuclear antibody, 69–70
Arthritis impact measurement scale, 21
Autoantibodies, 69–71
    anti-double-stranded-DNA antibody, 70
    antineutrophil cytoplasmic antibody, 70
    antinuclear antibody, 69–70
Azathioprine, 32–3

B
Bacterial septic arthritis, 83–4
Bath ankylosing spondylitis disease activity index, 21
Bath ankylosing spondylitis functional activity index, 21
Behçet's disease, 68
Biological agents, 36–7
Blood forms, 24
Brucellosis, 84
Buprenorphine, 28
Bursitis, 15, 51

C
Carpal tunnel syndrome, 49–50
Chondromalacia, 15
Churg-Strauss syndrome, 82
Ciclosporin, 34–5
Clinic checklist, 17
Codeine, 27
Cold agglutinins, 71
Complementary therapy, 26
Computed tomography, 20
Connective tissue diseases, 69–82
    anti-phospholipid syndrome, 75
    autoantibodies, 69–71
    differential diagnosis, 59, 79–80
    mixed connective tissue disease, 75
    polymyositis/dermatomyositis, 78–9
    Raymaud's phenomenon, 71–2
    scleroderma, 78
    Sjögren's syndrome, 76–7
    systemic lupus erythematosus, 72–4
Corticosteroids
    injections, 38–9
    rheumatoid arthritis, 62
Costochondritis, 14
Cryoglobulins, 70–1
Crystal arthritis, 90–2
    differential diagnosis, 59
    gout, 90–1
    pseudogout, 92
CT see Computed tomography
Cyclophosphamide, 35–6

D
Dactylitis, 13
De Quervain's tenosynovitis, 13, 52
Dermatomyositis, 78–9
DEXA see Dual energy X-ray absorptiometry
Dextropropoxyphene, 27
Diffuse idiopathic skeletal hyperostosis, 57
Dihydrocodeine, 27

NOTES

NOTES

NOTES

NOTES

Lightning Source UK Ltd.
Milton Keynes UK
UKOW050422240112

185940UK00001B/67/P